Robin Elizabeth is an Australian writer, ranter, reviewer, dyslexic, twitter addict, and definitely a mad mumma. She does enjoy getting caught in the rain, but not as much as she likes piña coladas and any number of 80s classic cocktails. Her friends have likened her to the comedian Judith Lucy, but no reputable source has confirmed the similarity. She is best known for her blog entries about postnatal depression and her support of the Australian publishing industry. She is known as a good literary citizen and has started *Robinpedia*, which humorously catalogues the ins and outs of the Australian writing industry.

Sunny Sydney is where Robin Elizabeth resides with her three children and a husband; not that she's entirely sure he exists because she only sights him but rarely. The children have been declared adorable by multiple sources.

http://riedstrap.wordpress.com

@RobinElizabee

https://facebook.com/confessionsofamadmooer

Confessions of a Mad Mooer
Postnatal Depression Sucks

Robin Elizabeth

Published by Bookends Publishing
Sydney Australia
http://bookendspublishing.com.au

First published by Bookends Publishing in 2016

Copyright held by Robin Elizabeth 2016

The moral right of the author has been asserted.

All rights reserved. No part of this book may be reproduced or transmitted by any person or entity, including internet search engines or retailers, in any form or by any means, electronic or mechanical, including photocopying (except under the statutory exceptions of the Australian Copyright Act 1968, recording, scanning or by any information storage and retrieval system without prior written permission of Robin Elizabeth.

ISBN-13: 978-0-646-59746-1

Cover image and design by Sally Walsh, Sillier than Sally Designs
Cover image and design copyright of Robin Elizabeth
Printed in Australia through IngramSpark
Print on demand for Amazon customers through CreateSpace

No antidepressants were harmed during the making of this book.

The content of this book is purely my opinion at the time of typing and should not be taken in place of professional medical or psychological advice. This is simply my story told my way at the time of writing it.

With thanks to Margie, Lesley, Helen and Lisa.

Strong and capable women
who make me a better person every day.

Contents

Confessions of a Mad Mooer 1
It's Okay if You Haven't Read or Watched *Girl, Interrupted*.. 7
My Oprah Moment 12
ALWAYS BACK UP YOUR SHIT 18
I Think I Agreed to Wear a Pirate Shirt............................. 21
Wabi-sabi and the Mona Lisa's Smile................................ 33
Carrots, Potatoes, and Broccoli....................................... 38
Girl Tribe 44
Invisible Prejudices... 57
The Charlotte Dawson Effect 66
Treat Yourself like a Friend.. 80
I'm an Arsehole Parent 91
The Mad Robin in the Attic 108
Play to Your Strengths.. 116
Impractical Parenting 129
Life Hacks for Women with PND 149
Memoir from the Madhouse 169
Other Titles by Robin Elizabeth 186
About Bookends Publishing.. 187

Confessions of a Mad Mooer

In April of 2014, I found myself in a psychiatric hospital. Not because I was visiting a sick relative but because I had gone completely around the bend. I had a two-year-old little girl and four-month-old identical twin boys. I'd had a rough entry to 2014 with the twins coming eight weeks early, me being diagnosed with high-grade abnormal cells in my fanwah, a weeklong trip to the hospital with my ever reoccurring pancreatitis, and then my baby boys ended up in hospital with breathing problems due to bronchiolitis. I was sleep-deprived, I was physically depleted from illness, I was anxious, and I could no longer cope. The doctors in the children's ward, on seeing how distressed I was, immediately referred me to one of the hospital's social workers, who in turn referred me to one of the hospital's psychiatrists. They said there was no doubt of the diagnosis; I had postnatal depression, or postpartum depression as they call it in the US, and I had it bad. It was suggested that heading off to a psychiatric hospital with a Mother and Baby unit that would take me and my boys was for the best. As soon as the twins were well enough to leave the hospital, the three of us were shipped off in order for me to begin intensive therapy.

I dealt with this turn of events the only way I knew how: through my writing. A couple of weeks into my stay, in what my fellow *inmates* and I came to lovingly term *the madhouse*, I began to blog about my experiences. My usual audience must have been slightly surprised by the sudden switch from sharing my fantasy stories and expressing my love of words, especially "bum," to writing about madness, but they thankfully went along with it and encouraged me to keep going. And so it was on the 1st of May 2014 that I wrote my very first entry about my journey through postnatal depression:

Hi, I'm a Mad Mooer

So it happened. I've gone completely around the bend. Had a nervous breakdown, got postnatal depression, had a meltdown, chucked a wobbly, got myself in a tizzy, whatever you want to call it. I've been a bit of a cow, and I'm mad. I've evidently got mad cow disease. I'm currently in the nuthouse. Or should I say, "I'm convalescing in a supportive medical environment whilst I recuperate from exhaustion."

And who wouldn't be exhausted with newborn twins and a toddler? Who wouldn't need help under these circumstances? Well, one of my cousins, for one, managed not to turn into a jibbering mess when she had a two year old plus newborn twins. And in my mind, everyone else in these circumstances sailed right on through except for me. At three months, I cracked it. I just cried and cried and cried and cried a bit more. My body hurt from trying to settle premature twins, born at 32 weeks and home from the NICU at 35 weeks, who never wanted to sleep. My brain hurt from trying to juggle my three babies. And my heart hurt from feeling as if I was failing all three of my children simultaneously. I couldn't get my twins to settle, and ended up spending so much time with them that I felt like my toddler was missing out. On top of that, if one twin had been crying for ninety minutes straight, I was to exhausted from dealing with him that I didn't have time for his brother when he inevitably started his round of crying.

What did I do? I kept telling the husband that I was exhausted, I couldn't cope, I needed help, and I couldn't do it any longer. He told me to "crack on," as it was only a tough phase; in a year's time, it'd all settle down, and I just needed to ride the wave. Turns out I don't know how to surf. Not even bodyboard, or boogie board, as it used to be called. Heck, I can't even body surf. To be perfectly honest, I don't even know if I can swim at this stage. (I know what you're thinking: can she stretch this metaphor any further? Surely not. Let dead horses lie, don't whip sleeping dogs, and, oh yeah, I can stretch it further.) It was like I'd been paddling in a kids' wading pool and all of a sudden had been thrown into the middle of an ocean, during a storm at night, with only one oar and nothing else to help me. Sure, an oar is useful when there is also a row boat and another oar, but when it's by itself, it just drags you down. My husband's pep talks, his delusional attempts at blind optimism, simply dragged me down further rather than helping me to rise to the occasion. With added support, I may very well have been able to rise to the occasion with his encouragement.

But there wasn't any, and I just sank deeper and deeper into depression until all three of my children got sick—joys of having a toddler in childcare: they bring every plague home, and I ended up in hospital with my little boys who had developed bronchiolitis from their sister's cold. After I'd just gotten out of hospital myself for pancreatitis, I lost it. I couldn't cope. When the paediatricians began their rounds I began sobbing uncontrollably. By coincidence, one of the doctors on rotation had been my daughter's paediatrician during her reflux and hip dysplasia. He saw me, could see how bad I had gotten, and immediately referred me to the hospital social worker, who referred me to the psychiatric team. So in turn I got referred to a Mother and Baby unit at a psychiatric hospital to get my bearings, physically recover, and try to sort through some stuff in my head.

How's it all going now? Well, I can tell you that inside my head is a terrifying place to be, but I'll keep you updated with my progress through more *Confessions of a Mad Mooer.*

This book deals with my thoughts about my journey through postnatal depression or, possibly more correctly, being diagnosed with depression postnatally. It includes some of my past blog entries on depression along with new, previously unshared material. So kick back, relax, and enjoy my random rantings about being a *Mad Mooer.*

It's Okay if You Haven't Read or Watched *Girl, Interrupted*

On the day I was to enter the psychiatric hospital, I tearfully told my husband that I hadn't even had time to watch *Girl, Interrupted* to prepare. How could I possibly be ready to hang out with a bunch of crazy ladies if I hadn't recently watched a movie about a bunch of crazy ladies? He said he felt that I would be okay. I cried anyway. I asked him if he was going to leave me in there forever. He comfortingly told me that he couldn't do that; the boys had to leave by the time they turned one at the latest. I asked him if he still loved me. He thankfully said yes, although he did sigh and roll his eyes at the question. I cried some more. I wasn't even in the hospital, and I already missed my daughter. Apart from the odd trip to the hospital for my dud pancreas, I had never been separated from her. I couldn't imagine a day without her, let alone weeks. I hugged her to me like a rag doll, never wanting to let her go. And I guess I was sad because I might miss my husband as well; he goes all right, I guess.

All the same, I still had to enter the hospital, despite being woefully underprepared. I hadn't seen *Sucker Punch* recently either. What if lobotomies were on offer? How on Earth would I know how to plan an escape without recently having watched *Terminator 2*? These were very real concerns.

Now I should probably make it very clear from the outset that psychiatric hospitals are nowhere near as exciting as they appear to be in movies. They're not even close. This is a point that I will repeatedly harp on about because I found it so shockingly different. It was both disappointing and comforting. Nobody is stealing guitars to serenade each other, nobody is sneaking off to have sex with orderlies, and most notably, nobody is hiding chicken carcasses under their bed. I was not the only patient who was hoping to catch someone out doing that. Chicken carcasses became a bit of a running joke. However, despite the distinct lack of avian skeletons, there are a few similarities. You do have a communal window where you have to line up for your meds, and there is group therapy, but they don't check under your tongue to make sure you've taken your medication, and group therapy is not exciting. Useful, yes; exciting, no. I cannot express to you just how different it is from the movies. It is depressingly civilised.

Now of course my concerns were irrational and in hindsight just a stalling tactic because nothing is ever like it is in the movies. The Mother and Baby unit was segregated from the rest of the hospital. We had our own little area and rooms with plenty of space for cots and toys, with their own bathrooms, televisions, and double beds. Our partners were even able to stay over every now and then for a bit of way-hey-hey in said double beds. The walls were all clean, the nurses weren't all scowling—well one bitch was, but you can't please everyone; you're not a cannoli donut—and I didn't even see an orderly, let alone one dragging a screaming patient away for daring to refuse medication. I think that the most exciting thing that I saw at the medication window was that one woman needed two signatures for her medication because it was particularly high grade. I was a bit jealous. The whole unit looked like a clean, if not a little dull, hotel. There was even a communal playroom for the kids, a large lounge room with the biggest television I have seen, and there was also a kitchen. A kitchen that had knives. We were entrusted to be near knives. And they weren't even corked. The patients roaming about were all wearing their own clothes and chatting calmly whilst playing with their babies. They all looked normal. They all seemed, dare I say it, pleasant.

I was simultaneously disappointed and relieved. I probably wouldn't have to make my own shank and fight off some deranged lunatic trying to kill or kidnap my babies, but it certainly wasn't going to be exciting enough to inspire a brilliant piece of writing like *One Flew Over the*

Cuckoo's Nest. Had Hollywood steered me wrong all these years? Had novels misled me? Was I no closer to becoming the next Sylvia Plath... without the suicide?

I didn't have much time to process the disappointment because my husband was leaving because he needed to get to work, and then I got my period for the first time since the twins were born. And to be perfectly honest, I was pretty pissed off about that too. Breastfeeding was supposed to guarantee no periods. It hadn't worked for my daughter, and yet again, they were back whilst I was still breastfeeding twins. The news was almost as bad as the fact that I was in the nuthouse and wouldn't be able to see my little girl every day.

Well, at least I still had my boys, I reasoned. Even with depression, and thoughts of ending my own life, I loved them utterly. They were so cute, and so smiley. A Colgate commercial ready to happen once they grew teeth. They only had two problems, really. Severe reflux, which caused them pain, and the fact that they wouldn't sleep. Unfortunately, even though there were only two problems, they were both utterly maddening. Every time my boys cried, the bile would rise in my own throat. They were suffering, and I wasn't mothering well enough to stop it. I felt that I had to solve everything that went wrong with them. I thought that it was all up to me, and that if I didn't fix it, then they would end up with long-term psychological damage. And of course whilst I tended to them, I felt as if I was neglecting my little girl who had been my sole focus for the past two years. No matter what I did, I was deeply scarring at least one of my children because I just wasn't good enough.

I blamed myself for everything. My children needed more, and I couldn't give it to them. Of course I now know what was needed was actual support for myself and that I wasn't doing anything wrong. Taking care of three kids under three years old on your own whilst your husband works ridiculously long hours is untenable, if not a little cruel. But at the time, I felt like an utter failure, even though objectively, I'd actually done really well despite contending with so many medical issues of my own.

I asked a total stranger for some pads and made a new friend in the process. She was nice. The woman didn't just give me one but a whole bunch. She seemed like a really kind, generous person who was great with their baby. The kind of mother that you see playing with her kid in the park and wish you were like. I would never have picked her as having postnatal depression. And of course, they would have thought the same thing about me. We were all just trying to do our best, often in impossible circumstances. Group therapy helped me realise this. As I've said, it wasn't as exciting as they depict in the movies, but it did help.

My Oprah Moment

Much of the treatment in the Mother and Baby unit focused around group therapy, so that's generally where I had my biggest breakthroughs. Even though I spent the first week in the madhouse so bitterly disappointed with the fact that it was nowhere near as entertaining as it "should" be, based on my Hollywood viewing experience it was still beneficial. Sure, nobody from group therapy tried to crawl into bed with me, and nobody stood up in the middle of therapy screaming, but it was still worthwhile. I mean, obviously it would have been better if we'd bonded together as a team and plotted our dramatic escape, but it was okay, I guess.

As a writer I was expecting to experience something exciting to write about. You know, come up with the next *Bell Jar*. Some dramatic confessions, arguments, the odd chair thrown and, of course, being that we're all women, the obligatory catfight that devolves into a group pillow fight. Totally did not happen. Not even close. The closest we got was someone saying I had no filter between my mind and my mouth. I had to agree, so no animosity, backstabbing, or pillow fighting ensued.... Okay, I do think she was a bit of a bitch, but I didn't verbalise it at the time. I'll take care of that now. *Bitch!* See how much I have matured from all the therapy?

In group therapy you sit in a circle, yes, like the movies, but you get manuals. You pause thoughtfully as you try to articulate how the theory relates to yourself personally, but not too personally—no sordid tales or juicy titbits, really—can't have us getting too excited. One woman got into trouble for sharing too much information about her ex, even though it didn't involve anything too smexy. Perhaps that was the problem. The therapist was all like, "If I have to hear one more of your inane stories about your deadbeat ex, it better at least have some sex in there." Anyway, getting back to appropriate behaviour, you nod supportively when another person is speaking to show that, yes, you understand them and appreciate their comments and feelings. You don't threaten to strangle others or kill yourself. It's all very civilised. It's more like a group of girls out to coffee but with guided conversation and more thoughtful pauses. *Le sigh*, not the stuff of a best-selling novel with a spin-off blockbuster film. I guess I could sex it up a bit. Put in a lesbian love triangle and then the struggle to return to heterosexual family life, and yet somehow be only nineteen instead of in my mid-thirties... *Sucker Swan... Brokeback, Interrupted*??? I'll work on it. There's something there, once I put in some forced drug use and us all wearing flimsy white hospital gowns, that somehow get wet, instead of our own clothes... Send me an e-mail with some suggestions; we'll crowd write it. Anyway, back to my point: group therapy is not the awesomely hilarious experience you see in comedies. Just be warned about that. Don't get your hopes up on the therapist who clearly has more issues than anyone else, or alcoholics and sexually promiscuous over-sharers. They aren't there.

I'd been convalescing for about three weeks when the penny really dropped for me. In group therapy, we'd been looking at Cognitive Behavioural Therapy, or CBT for those up on the lingo. It basically looks at how we respond to an event. How what we think, often unnecessarily negatively, effects how we respond to a situation and therefore how we feel and act, and then the consequences of that. Makes sense, right? A common example used for mothers is, the baby is crying. Then you list what your thoughts are about it. For me that starts with, "the baby is crying because something is wrong." I then ramp up to, "I'm doing something wrong—I'll never do this right, my babies will be permanently damaged because I'm not responding right—I am the worst mother of all time—if I could just do this right, my baby wouldn't be crying—I am ruining my children's lives with my incompetence—I may as well die... in a toilet... with no friends and nobody loving me. I suck." As a consequence, I get stressed. Simple, really.

The madhouse wasn't the first place that I had encountered CBT. I am a big fan of Martin Seligman and have read all of his books. They outline CBT quite clearly. Logically, I already understood this. It was easy for me to do that exercise and a range of other scenarios because I totally get that I'm a great big pessimist. Sadly, my emotions were running rings around me. Being able to complete those exercises and understand I was catastrophising wasn't stopping me from feeling utterly like shit. But then, three weeks in, we had a different group-therapy leader, and she said something a little bit different. When we got to stating our thoughts/beliefs about the situation, the therapist said, "Now how does that relate to your core beliefs about yourself?" And the world went CLICK. Suddenly I was forced to think about what I truly thought about myself deep down. And that my beliefs and reactions to all these different situations all stem from one underlying core belief.

I didn't have multiple problems, but just one giant problem—this very horrible and very misguided notion I have about myself. So here's what I wrote all in a rush as the emotional floodgates opened—*I can't do anything right, I poison everything I touch, I'm not good enough, I'm not enough enough, I am a bad person, I don't deserve to be happy, I deserve to be punished, I am garbage, I AM AN*

EVIL PIECE OF SHIT. And then it was as if a huge ray of sunshine broke free, and I just smiled. I wrote down all those awful things I believe about myself, and all I felt was elation and happiness because it meant that I knew where my problems lay.

It is now two years later, and I am far from perfect, but I now have more of a chance of halting the escalation of my anxiety because I know it comes from within me, within my own self-loathing psyche, not from an event, person, or situation. I don't need to conquer a myriad of thoughts regarding a thousand different events; I need to conquer myself and essentially one thought, which is *I'm not good enough to exist.* It is exceptionally hard work and a long journey to rid myself of this core belief that has been ground into me through my entire childhood. However, finally in 2014, at the age of 34, I had found a map of where to start. Sure, I'm discovering that some of the streets are misnamed and some roads have closed, but at least I have found myself a start and an end point. And that has been invaluable. I constantly have to remind myself that I'm not a bad person, that it's just a difficult situation, not because of me, but just because it is. Everything bad in the world is not my fault; I just hate myself and think that it is. It is liberating, even though it is awful. I highly recommend examining your core belief about yourself. What do you really think about yourself?

Confessions of a Mad Mooer

How do you explain to yourself good and bad things? It will horrify you and then set you free.

ALWAYS BACK UP YOUR SHIT

I need you to know that as I was just typing this up, the first draft that is. Don't worry—I got an editor. I'm dyslexic; I know you don't want to be wading through my stuff and looking at beautiful descriptions of azure qlue water and be thinking, "Qlue, what the F is QLUE?!" only to find out I meant blue. Anyway, as I was typing up the first draft of *Mad Mooer*, I got a little bit carried away and hadn't been paying attention to my battery life. I typed, full of empowered glory, "It will horrify you and then set you free." BLANK SCREEN. The battery conked out. I let out a scream like Ned Flanders seeing a set of purple drapes and began to hyperventilate. I ran from my bedroom, where I'd been working completely naked, for reasons I don't even understand, and started madly fumbling around in front of an open window, desperately trying to pull my charger out of a box. Caught sight of a neighbour. I awkwardly dragged the box where my chargers are to the floor and crumpled down behind it to hide my shame and continued searching for my laptop charger. I finally found it making love to other electrical cords and not wanting to be disturbed. It initially refused to come with me. I managed to coax it away from its multiple lovers, plugged it into my computer, and all was fine. Everything was still there.

Now I may have overreacted just a smidgen, but the reason is because in August of last year, just before I was about to send parts three and four of *What Happens in Book Club...* to my editor, my laptop died. It DIED! Not in a, "oh, don't worry; we can get your data back," way; it died in a, "you've lost everything, everything, EVERYTHING!!! Thank goodness you're so lazy that you never delete your photos off your camera because at least you still have all your kids' photos because you have to resave them because everything, including your precious books, are *GONE*," kind of way. That is my least favourite way. After which, I fell into a very deep depression and basically couldn't write much for a long time. I was just empty.

People like to glorify depression and link it to the creative process. They believe that it helps you write. It doesn't. True, clinical depression, disconnects you from your feelings. You simply do not have access to the emotions necessary for writing. It's not just that you have writer's block; you have life block. Depression is not the same as being sad, or grieving, or having anxiety. All of those conditions you can write through very easily. Anxiety is my standard mode—trust me, you can write with it. Depression is a very different, and isolating, experience.

In retrospect, I realise that my reaction to this data loss was pretty stupid. Like, seriously: how hard is it to rewrite stuff that you've already written? It really shouldn't be difficult. In fact, if I was a go-getting optimist, I would have seen it as an opportunity to write something even better, but I didn't. I just wallowed like... something that wallows a lot.

My advice to you, if you are anxious, and even if you are not—always save your work to three different devices, place a protection spell over your laptop, keep sage in your underpants, and pray to at least seven different deities, in order to ensure you don't lose your precious data. I had done none of these things and was left with nothing. And yes, I was formerly a high school teacher, and I went through university, so I know the importance of backing things up. But I didn't. You're probably wondering why. Because I'm crazy. Haven't you been reading? And yes, I blamed myself for being a complete loser/idiot who must secretly want to sabotage her life for not backing up her files because that's what anxious people do. But, over a year later, I am just about recovered, and writing more productively again. It doesn't matter how many times you fall, as long as you get up one more time than you fall. Fuck, that was an inspiring sentence.

I Think I Agreed to Wear a Pirate Shirt

Full disclosure: I didn't find every single part of my stay in the chicken coup helpful. It wasn't just a series of lightbulb moments between brushing other ladies' hair, having tickle fights, and singing sweet lullabies to peaceful babies. To be perfectly frank, I loathed my first week in the psychiatric hospital with the intensity of a thousand suns. It sucked balls.

During my first week in hospital, I have never contemplated suicide more often in my life, and I've been contemplating suicide since I was four, so I've done a lot of contemplating in my time. Initially, you are thrust into this unfamiliar environment, with strangers. This is an introvert's worst nightmare. Sure, those strangers are either fellow *inmates* suffering from the exact same condition as you or are trained professionals, but they don't know you. You don't know your fellow crazies well enough to trust them yet, which you do completely by the time you leave (shout out to my girls; let's have some chicken soon), and the medical staff doesn't know you well enough to support you yet. I wasn't the only one who hated my first week. One woman even packed up her shit and left on the first night. I reiterate: it sucks balls to begin with. Bear with it. It gets better.

For the first two nights that you are there, the nurses take your baby at nighttime so that you can sleep. Sounds like heaven, right? Wrong. Because you don't get to sleep through the night. You get woken up and asked if you want to feed the baby. Even if you have left expressed breastmilk and bottles with them, you are still woken and asked. Sure, you don't have to resettle them, but it isn't exactly ideal if you need real rest. Two lots of six or, better yet, eight hours of sleep would be amazing. It would have done wonders. I didn't get that once while I was in hospital. The most I ever got was four hours. This, ironically, was on nights that the twins were with me and not the nurses.

I went into the psychiatric hospital in bad shape. I had suffered through pancreatitis less than a month earlier. The treatment is NIL by mouth, which means you cannot eat or drink anything, not even water. Which as you can imagine, is heaps of fun when you're breastfeeding twins. Then I was in hospital tending to the boys with their respiratory problems. I recognise that I may have been more worn-out than the hospital was used to dealing with, but still, they had my records, and... we were all fucking exhausted. Not just me. Depression is exhausting; newborns are exhausting. Even without adding debilitating pancreatitis and twins, all the mums there were exhausted, so you'd think something a little more beneficial than an interrupted two nights would be on offer. When I complained to one of the nurses that being woken up wasn't very helpful, I got told to stop talking rubbish, that the night nurses weren't "stupid;" they knew that the two nights were for rest and would not be waking anyone. Lesson learned, I never asked that nurse for help again. I had never thought that the night nurses were doing it because they were "stupid" but because it was, for some reason, policy. I was hoping it could be changed. Obviously not, with that nurse's attitude. And quite frankly, every other patient had whinged about it too, so this nurse must have been off her own meds that day... or she's just a manky ho—who knows? I had mostly positive experiences with the rest of the nurses. I would hate to tar them all with the same manky brush. Many were straight-up angels, but there's always one, isn't there? I guess you can't have heroes without having a few villains.

Because I had twins, I actually got offered three nights of baby minding up front. Don't get too excited. It's not as if they take them 7pm to 7am; it's more like 10:30pm to 6am, which would still be awesome if you didn't get woken up repeatedly. On the third day, when my fellow *inmates* found out that I had been given three nights, they lost their shit. And to my surprise, not at me.

They weren't angry at me for getting a night extra, they were angry because they felt that I should be given more. Yep, those crazy bitches were amazing. They had my back. They said I deserved at least four nights, two nights per baby, and then some extra nights thrown in because I had been so ill. I couldn't believe it. I had never before in my life been in an environment where people wanted to give me extra. To say I was touched would be an understatement. I couldn't express my gratitude at the time because I was so crazy from sleep deprivation that nothing was entering into my brain or coming out of it very well, but I hope they all knew how grateful I was. My husband also rang up the nurses and spoke with them about my illnesses and my exhaustion and reminded them of the hospital report that they had on me, and would they mind catering to my individual circumstances as the hospital had said they would before I was admitted? They agreed. We started doing a rotation of me handing the boys over every second to third night at 11pm and them coming back to me at 6am. The nurses still woke me though. Just not every three hours. And generally to ask me if I was sleeping okay. Old habits die hard, I guess.

Even when I had the twins in with me, the nurses still woke me up. At nighttime, they have to do their rounds. You know, make sure we haven't escaped, murdered our babies, or started stuffing chicken carcasses under fellow *inmates*' beds. So every damn time they entered, you'd hear the loud sucking noise of the "soundproofing" around the doors followed by the flash of the torch. Some of my fellow *inmates* had developed elaborate fantasies about stealing the torch and replacing it with a smaller, softly lit one. Clearly, we weren't the criminally insane type, when our wildest fantasies involved theft and replacement, but those lights were super annoying. It was like being invaded by the secret police in the middle of the night repeatedly. I was willing to confess to anything to make them stop coming for me, but unfortunately, I didn't know if they were after communists, Nazis, or witches, so didn't know whom to throw under the bus. Most women began draping cloths over their doors to stop the sucking noise being so loud. I tried it—the noise was still plenty loud. I guess it was yet another metaphor for our lives: you suck just as much as this sucky door. Ouch.

    I remember one such nighttime raid vividly. The boys had been super restless that night. I'd had one or the other in my bed with me all night as I became too exhausted to either rock or pat them and would collapse into bed with a warm little body next to mine. I was constantly exchanging babies as one drifted off and the other then stirred, so it was all becoming a bit of a blur as to which baby was which. But finally, all three of us had managed to doze off. One baby was in his own little crib, the other snuggled up next to me, when I heard the inevitable sucking noise and the flash of light. I kept my eyes closed, hoping that this time, they wouldn't speak to me, and I could just sleep. But the light piercing through my closed eyelids didn't go away. The nurse was lingering in there, and then I heard rummaging. I sat up at this point. I was wondering why the fuck nurses would be going through my shit—trust me, I had nothing exciting that they'd want; I hadn't even packed a razor, for fear they'd view it as a weapon. The nurse then turned the flashlight full into my face, and I heard a very angry, "Where's the baby, Robin?" My heart lurched into my throat. One of my babies was missing. I instantly wanted to vomit. "Is he gone?" I asked, hysterical. "There's only one here," the angry reply came. Then she flashed the torch at my peaceful angel in his crib, and he began to stir. I stared at the nurse, dumbfounded, and pointed at the baby right next to me. She'd missed a baby that wasn't at all hidden. I'd slept without a blanket and pillow because I was paranoid that I might snuffle him. Worst of all, both babies woke up. The nurse simply nodded, then left. She didn't help to resettle the babies that she had awoken, just woke everyone, and then pissed off. I was not happy. Nobody enjoyed the nighttime raids, especially not my babies. So, should you find yourself convalescing in a supportive medical environment, might I suggest to you that you pack earplugs and an eye mask? You'll need them.

To top off the stress of continued sleep deprivation and getting used to a new environment, I was put on lockdown for the first week of my stay in the facility. This is possibly what made my first week so challenging. On entering the hospital, patients are given a few surveys to fill out. One is the standard K10 test, which everyone has failed spectacularly before entering anyway, and others are more specific. I had answered yes to "thinking about suicide" on these forms. Big mistake, huge; the nurses freaked and said I couldn't go anywhere. The Mother and Baby unit is pretty chill, unless it is group or meal time, you are pretty much free to walk around the neighbourhood with your baby—or babies, in my case. I, on the other hand, couldn't go. A little known fact about me is that not only am I a high school teacher, but I'm also a fully qualified personal trainer. I actually enjoy physical activity. The hospital, which now has a gym, didn't at the time; I wasn't allowed to take the boys out, and I was trapped inside. I began to get cabin fever. I longed for fresh air, I longed to stretch my legs, and I longed for my boys to actually be able to get some sun and vitamin D. I simply couldn't cope. I was going completely bonkers, and I knew being cooped up was making my condition worse, so after five days, I simply lied and said I no longer thought about suicide and was allowed off house arrest. With more sleep and being allowed out, I improved rapidly. I could actually apply lessons that I had learned in group therapy and not just rock and jibber.

I'm not recommending that people lie on their questionnaires. Just letting people know the consequences of my answer. It hadn't occurred to me for a moment that saying yes to having suicidal thoughts would be considered a big deal in that environment. I kind of assumed everyone was feeling suicidal, or why else would they be there? The fact that people would get themselves admitted prior to being suicidal was not a notion that I had even entertained. To be honest, when people tell me they have never considered suicide, I always just assume they're lying. The idea that their life has not ever sucked hard enough to want to end it all is just foreign to me, so the fact that I was banned from accessing fresh air for something that I considered to be fairly normal surprised me. It was the only time in my life when I had considered suicide for a reason other than thinking I was such a burden on others that they'd be better off without me. I actually started wanting to commit suicide inside the facility just to show the staff how stupid they were for thinking keeping me inside could stop someone from killing themselves. There are endless ways I could have killed myself whilst inside their very own walls; keeping me away from sunlight and fresh air was patently stupid as far as I was concerned. I do realise that they had liability and had to take some action, but it was a very dangerous action for someone such as myself, who finds physical activity important.

Not only did I desire activity, but I wanted alone time. Not necessarily alone time away from my boys—I was happy to go walking with them—but alone time away from the facility. I needed some distance from the drone of the system. I have always liked to recharge my batteries alone in quiet, dimly lit spaces. Walking at dusk is great for me. Low light, crisp fresh air, the universe, and me. It's like a brain clean and body recharge in one. As soon as I was able to get out and walk my boys and be alone with the quiet of my thoughts at dusk, I began to feel much better. I nearly cried with joy on my first excursion out to a nearby park. It became a much needed part of my healing, walking through the park as the world turned from day to night and allowing that dichotomy to inspire me. I'm not sure how I would have coped if I had been kept inside any longer. The urge for suicide was very strong. I had to seriously weigh up the damage I would do to my kids by them not having a mother and her taking her own life versus the damage of having a depressed mother in their life. In the end, I decided that a violent death would be more destructive, but I'm not sure I could have maintained that stance for another week. Air and sunshine are important; they aren't a cure, but denial of them can be catastrophic.

Not only did I hate my first week in the psychiatric hospital—yes, I know hate is a strong word, but it is appropriate in this case—but I also got nothing out of my meetings with my psychiatrist. Well, I got antidepressants, that was good, but apart from that, it seemed to be of little use to me. Plenty of women in there loved their psychiatrists, and admittedly, nobody else had the same person that I did, so it could be just me, or just the person assigned to me, or a combination of us, but I got nothing out of it... except for the drugs.

Seeing the psychiatrist appointed to me by the hospital was somewhat complicated by the fact that he was a low talker. By that, I don't mean he had a deep voice. I mean he spoke so quietly that I couldn't understand most of what he said. After leaving the facility, I actually met someone who had this same person appointed to them. They apparently walked out of their very first session and demanded a new person because how the heck could they get better if they couldn't hear a damned word he said? They were duly assigned a new doctor. I wish I had been that confident because the other women there raved about their psychiatrists. They had meetings, their husbands were called in to discuss issues, their parents were even called in, and they worked through problems. It sounded magnificent. Kind of what you'd expect from therapy.

My therapist was not so magnificent for me. Mine spoke so softly I could barely gain the gist of what was said. I knew my medication was being increased to a "therapeutic" level and that they'd like to put me on certain other medications; however, I'd have to stop breastfeeding to take it, so that wasn't going to work very well for me. I asked him if he wanted to meet my husband, and he said no and that it was "interesting" that I would ask him that. I said I asked because the other patients were doing that with their psychiatrists, and he then asked me why I didn't go to coffee with the other women. It was two other women who went for coffee, not all the other women. I simply shrugged as my answer. I should have told him that I was exhausted, that I kind of had twins and was recovering from pancreatitis, and nobody else was doing that. But thanks for making me feel like I'm totally antisocial, you a-hole. Not that it bothered me. I'm totes okay with it. Totes. You know that someone really means it when they say "totes." I went to the mandatory psychiatric sessions. Ticked off those boxes, but it wasn't for me. I did request to see a psychologist, but they felt nobody would have the time... Make time. It's a fucking psychiatric hospital—what else are they doing?

When my husband asked me what my psychiatrist was like, I simply responded with, "I don't know, but I'm pretty sure that I just agreed to wear a pirate shirt." Being an avid Seinfeld fan, he understood exactly what I meant.

He looked forward to the day the psychiatrist would chase me from the room, screaming, "Motherfucker." Unfortunately, as I keep on telling you, it isn't like the movies, and nothing that exciting happens in there.

Wabi-sabi and the Mona Lisa's Smile

Talk about being a negative Nancy! I had better turn this thing around with some positive Polly, because although individual sessions with my psychiatrist were a calamitous failure—or should I say *murmuring* failure?—and I hated my first week, I did quite surprise myself by enjoying art therapy. I'll be perfectly honest: I was not initially impressed on seeing that I was being forced to do art therapy. I was all like, "But I'm a writer; don't you people have writing as therapy? Can't I skip the art therapy classes and just sit and write?" The nurses were all like, "No." But it actually turned out to be good.

For those wondering what art therapy is, it's essentially a place where people who are good at art can draw/paint/create visual masterpieces that express their inner turmoil or longed-for optimism, and the rest of the basket cases can just have fun doodling or making jewellery as if we were little kids again. In the nuthouse, I made three bracelets for my daughter. It was nice to have the distraction. Plus it helped allay my guilt for not being with her by at least being able to make her little gifts. Now that might not be the technical explanation of what art therapy is; I did try to research what it was (I posted on a friend's Facebook page, who teaches art therapy, "What do you do in art therapy?" I'm thinking investigative journalism may not be my thing) but I'm sure this gives the general gist.

I'll apologise in advance because things are about to get a little bit arty farty, but we are about to talk about art therapy, so that's to be expected.

Art therapy can be quite daunting the first time you do it. Thoughts race like, "What the fuck am I supposed to be doing? How can finger painting help me?" For those that are artistically inclined, the feelings are apparently much worse. Fears of creating imperfect work abound; anxiety over time constraints ensue, and before you know it, the artists have given up, started doodling, and are not creating the Sistine Chapel just like everyone else. Whatever your art level is, this foray into a new environment seems to bring out similar fears: *my work won't be perfect, I'm not perfect, I suck.*

It's interesting that we as mothers hold ourselves to such ridiculously high standards that a simple art class can dredge up such a tidal wave of self-doubt and loathing. We want to do our very best and our children's futures seem to be in peril with every decision that we make. Today's saturation of parenting experts and baby whisperers only make things worse. If you're not looking in your baby's eyes as they play, you're making them feel abandoned. Pretty hard if you've got twins and/or another child/children. Pretty hard even with just one baby if you need to go to the toilet, brush your teeth, or, heaven forbid, take a shower. If your baby cries, they are getting permanent brain damage. Again, toileting and showering becomes a guilt-ridden nightmare. If you just feed your baby enough and make them feel secure, they'll be settled and sleep well. An absolute guilt trip into crazy town that last one is.

This notion that if you do it "right," your baby will be happy and content is a crock. A baby is their own person, with their own thoughts, and their own needs. There will be times when their needs are way more complicated than feed, play, sleep. Even more complicated than adding a bath or wrapping or not wrapping or massaging or... or... or... or.... The list goes on. When these inevitable unsolvable fits of crying happen to a mother without postnatal depression, they get stressed and anxious. They then move on after the incident is over. When this happens to us mums with postnatal depression, we start to spiral out of control. Our baby is crying, and we can't stop the baby crying despite trying every trick in the book and writing a few new chapters; therefore, we are failing our baby. Our babies are going to become destitute, social misfits. Even worse, they're going to turn into the emotional cripples that we are. Our beautiful, perfect babies would be better off without us around to screw them up.

These catastrophic notions start to overwhelm us. Before you know it, we're out to sea, trying to use a pillow as a boat and a cap gun as an oar. Now I like cap guns and pillows as much as the next person, but they're not exactly the correct tools for getting by out at sea. Don't get me wrong—they're great. Please, don't slam me in the review section, saying "stop pillow shaming." I'm just saying there's a time and a place. A pillow is a fail as an oar. Just like expecting to be so perfectly in tune with your babies that they are always smiling or sleeping soundly is a fail in reality. This idealisation of clinical perfection prevents us from being in the moment. It stops us from appreciating our experience as beautiful despite the "flaws" because, deep down, we are so ashamed of ourselves for not living up to these expectations of perfection that we can barely breathe.

In art, there is a concept known as wabi-sabi. In a nutshell, wabi-sabi is the singular beauty in something that may first look wrong or flawed. It is the ability to see that the defects don't actually take away from the aesthetic but enhance it. If you think of a sunset, it isn't perfectly lined colours with a perfectly circular yellow sun in the middle. It's a miasma of colours with a globular orange sun slowly oozing downwards. This bleeding of warmth and colours is far more beautiful than if it was perfectly ruled lines on a page. Even in great art, the "flaws" are still there. The transient nature of the human condition was something that the great da Vinci strove to capture and did so most famously in his masterpiece, which we call *Mona Lisa*. He deliberately attempted to capture a smile that was dynamic and fleeting because that is what he saw when he walked the streets. He could see the beauty in this in-between moment, and evidently, we can too because people are still lining up to see her crooked smile. We can appreciate the imperfections in art; we can compose sonnets about it in nature, yet we condemn it in ourselves.

Sitting there mindlessly beading gave my brain a chance to relax. It gave me a moment to just stop spiralling and reset. I'm not that bad. I'm imperfect, as were the bracelets I made. But imperfect is okay. We all just need to embrace the wabi-sabi, be our own sunset, and be our own Mona Lisa's smile. Why be a cookie-cutter image when you can be complex, fine art?

Carrots, Potatoes, and Broccoli

Okay, that last section got a little heavy with the artistic wankatude. I apologise. I did a BA, so can get a little theoretical and heady at times. Let's bring it back down to reality with a chat about hospital food. I have spent extensive amounts of time in hospital. I have a dud pancreas, therefore from time to time, I end up in hospital on a cocktail of painkillers and NIL by mouth. When they ease you back onto food, to ensure you can eat without exploding from both ends and doubling over in pain, they put you on a clear-food diet. They tell you that this involves jelly, apple juice, and broth. This sounds kind of awesome. The only awesome part of this is the apple juice, which tastes like heaven after being denied food for sometimes weeks at a time. This desperation for food, unfortunately, cannot make hospital jelly or broth taste better. The jelly is vomitously sweet, and the broth isn't so much broth as Bonox and water. It tastes like bitterness and the ashes of destroyed dreams. Once you graduate from apple juice and refusing to eat jelly and "broth," you get "treated" to real hospital food. Just quietly, I'm fairly confident that hospitals save on money by serving up removed organs as protein. I'm pretty sure that I've had my own gallbladder served back to me and a few umbilical cords. When people say hospital food is bad, they're not exaggerating. Always order the sandwiches for lunch and dinner until they ban you. Fortunately, food at the psychiatric hospital was markedly better. Perhaps it's because they aren't performing organ removals so have to actually source their protein from outside the hospital grounds.

Given that I went into the psychiatric hospital on the back of two stays in regular hospital, the food was a welcome relief. It was real, it was hot, it wasn't wet, and it tasted reasonable. I was also able to go and eat it at a table rather than in my bed. It was almost like being human again. However, there was an element to the menu that soon began to drain on me. It was the accompaniment to every meal. Potatoes, broccoli, and crinkle-cut carrots. My relief at edible food soon faded to boredom and then heightened to horror as the weeks wore on. By week three I simply couldn't face another meal with potatoes, broccoli, and crinkle-cut carrots on the side. It got so bad that we all began joking that they must have put one of the OCD patients in the kitchen for some rehab. The head chef would walk in, all excited for the day. "Okay, guys, let's do something different today. I'm thinking an Italian theme. How about a little lasagne, maybe a nice Italian salad on the side?" And of course, we'd end up with lasagne with potatoes, broccoli, and carrots. The next day the head chef would come in and say, "Wooooohoooo, I'm coming down with Mexican fever today. Let's do some tacos, some homemade guacamole. It's going to be fantastic. You can do it, Frank." In the end, they plate up tacos with potatoes, broccoli, and carrots. "Time for Chinese food. Who doesn't love sang choi bow? Come on Frank, you can do some Asian greens, even include some Chinese broccoli." And so we crazies are served up sang choi bow with potatoes, broccoli, and carrots. "Seriously, Frank? You've shown no fucking progress; get your head out of your arse and serve something different." Ladies, here are you potatoes, broccoli, and crinkle cut fucking carrots.

I shouldn't be too hard on them. They're dealing with a lot of crazy people. Maybe if they gave us too much variety for our sides, we'd start getting ideas. They'd find us sitting nude in a janitor's cupboard reading poetry whilst smoking a kranjska. Can't have us going all *Dead Poets Society* on them. Particularly because none of our group therapists were inspiring enough to have us clambering up onto tables and declaring them our captain. One of my group leaders actually told me to just quit writing until the kids were all older. Robin Williams would NEVER have said that. It just wouldn't work at all.

Honestly, our biggest source of excitement was watching *MKR* and discussing the impending *Eurovision* finals. But even our enthusiasm over television shows was kept at bay by the rigid structure of our ward. The whole decor seemed to be designed to ensure we weren't too stimulated. The communal lounge room had square chairs, square coffee tables, rectangular rugs, and a giant rectangle flat-screen TV mounted on the wall. Very orderly. It's like the structured furnishings would help keep us calm so that we wouldn't go wild. Probably so that we wouldn't start making crazy demands like having something other than potatoes, broccoli, and carrots with every damn meal. In fact, if we giggled too loudly whilst watching our guilty evening pleasure of *MKR*, the nurses stared at us and asked us if we'd like our evening medication. Couldn't have us giggling too loudly; there's trouble to be had there—better medicate us and ship us off to bed. But I'm proud to say we persisted in rebelling. I even got a couple of magazines with sexy sealed-sections and left them in the communal area. Shhhhh, don't tell anyone it was me.

But even with all this structure, the staff couldn't diminish the untamed ecstasy that is *Eurovision*. Perhaps the hospital has better results further away from the finals. Because we tended to remain defiant and fobbed away our evening medication until we were told quite sternly that it was late, and the medication window would be closing, and *if we didn't take our freakin' meds right now,* we'd get reported to our psychiatrists. Given that mine was such a low talker that I wouldn't have been able to understand any lecture I received, this was possibly not such a great threat to use on me. Unfortunately, my compadres quite liked their psychiatrists *and* could understand every word that they said, so I had no allies to fight the power with. But we still talked big.

And as for *Eurovision* 2014, what a spectacular winner. Conchita Wurst. An Austrian drag queen with exquisite eyes, the voice of an angel, and a beard. A real "stuff you" to the establishment. A celebration of being unique. It showed that you can be different and not deficient. Just like myself and my fellow mums were. We were anxious, we were guilt ridden, and we were gradually getting hairier ourselves because most of us assumed that we wouldn't be allowed to bring in a razor, but we were great. We loved each other. We laughed with each other. We empowered each other in that "you're weird and I'm weird, but that's okay" kind of way. So as much as the food, the furniture, and the nurses wished we'd just mellow the fuck out a bit and follow an orderly life, it was the moments of joined rebellion that really helped get us through. It gave us a much needed sense of ourselves and let us know that we were still fun and good company. I still love those girls. I know you're reading this. You're possibly the only ones reading this. Big smooshy kisses to you all.

Looking back, there seems to be an awfully high correlation between *inmates* and a love of *Eurovision*. I'm not saying you have to be crazy to like it, but apparently, it helps. If you, like me and my crazy-arsed friends, find yourself getting the tingles each year as the *Eurovision* final approaches, then maybe you should consider getting yourself checked out. Personally, I think you're crazy if you don't like it. What's not to love? The wind, the glitter, the dancing, the miming. It's champagne television. But what would I know? I'm nuts.

Girl Tribe

These days, there's a big push to get yourself a girl tribe. Lots of articles have come out about how women who have strong female relationships have more life satisfaction than those who don't. Essentially being in this environment of all women forced us into a girl tribe. You might come from different suburbs, have totally different jobs, be from different ethnicities or religions, but you had two things in common. 1) You had at least one kid and 2) you were mental. Please note: if you haven't been in a psychiatric hospital, you probably shouldn't call us mental, or crazy, or any of those other names that I have been using liberally. We laugh when we do it, but it always comes across as mean or condescending if others do it. You have to walk the walk to talk the talk, so I'm afraid, unless you're willing to go check yourself in for help, you should probably just stick to calling us by our actual names. If that bothers you, you might need to think about why you want to call us names. It's not like you're claiming them back for empowerment purposes if you're using them against others.

When I first checked into hospital, I hated it there. I was exhausted. I didn't find the nurses as helpful as had been promised, and I felt pretty sorry for myself because my husband was too busy to visit often. I felt rejected and alone. I cried a lot, I texted him a lot, I was sad a lot. That's a lot of a lots. I even sent the husband a pic of myself in a T-shirt and underpants in an attempt to lust him into coming to the rescue. It didn't help that staff commented on how my husband lived so close, and they were therefore shocked he didn't come to visit me more often. I already felt bad enough without their confirmation that I had been utterly abandoned. But ironically, I came to see his absence as a blessing. I think it was one of the factors that helped me make real progress. Many of the women in there had similarly busy husbands, or husbands that lived hours away and couldn't duck in to see them and continue working to pay the rent and medical bills.

In the third week that I was in the hospital, a few women came in who had husbands who pretty much stayed with them the whole time. At first, I thought it was sweet, but then I started to see how it drained on those women and isolated them from some of the funner aspects, the not-medical aspects. Whilst we abandoned ladies sat up late gossiping and eating chocolate as if we were naughty teenagers, they had husbands to be with. We got to blow off steam and talk about how much we hated men and how all men sucked, which was important because of... reasons..., but their husbands were right there next to them, chewing, breathing, snoring, and farting. These women did not get a moment's peace to themselves whereas those of us there with just our kids had a real chance to focus on ourselves. To kick back, to bond, to bitch, to forget about bras and just be us. It was pretty magnificent. We got to not only connect with our babies but ourselves.

Some of my fondest memories actually come from conversations with the girls and not from therapy. And these moments never fail to make me smile when I remember them. Having a bunch of crazy women that I can shout out to when I do something weird, and that can make me feel normal by saying, "me too," is always helpful. All I have to do is say "chicken carcasses," and those girls get exactly what I mean. It's important to have people in your life who have seen you ugly cry, respond to questions with grunts, make incredibly sarcastic comments to medical staff, eat half of the sandwiches yourself, lose your shit because you missed out on sandwiches, and still love you. I'll add my voice to this popular movement and say, get yourself a girl tribe. Seriously, when you're bat-shit crazy, you need them for everything. And I mean everything.

I think when we get pregnant, we have these notions of perfect warm little creatures that we can cuddle and love. That it will be a bonding experience for not just us and the baby but the whole family. It's almost as if we're so full of love hormones that we think that they will flutter out to the rest of the world and cover it in a rosy glow. You only have to go online and check out a pregnancy forum to discover just how wrong that notion is. Online pregnancy groups are supposed to be a place where expectant mothers can come together and support each other. And yes, there is that element to it, but as you know, for every action, there is an opposite and equal reaction. And in the pregnancy world, that reaction is savage.

There seems to be a certain subset of women who have made it their life's mission to make you feel bad no matter what you say. *Oh, you're craving Maltesers? I only ever craved kelp in my pregnancy. Oh, you're not walking well towards the end of your pregnancy with twins? I guess some bodies just aren't cut out for pregnancy. I never had any problems with my singletons. Oh, you want to punch me in my stupid face? Your baby is going to grow up to be a serial killer because you've poisoned them with negative emotions in utero.* And unfortunately, it doesn't stop there. Once you've had your baby, or babies, then you may as well just slap on a label, *Hi, I'm a mother; please give me unsolicited advice.* Because no matter what you do as a mother, according to "sanctimommies" on the Internet, you are doing it wrong. In fact, let me tell you just a few ways that you suck, just in case, unlike me, you've had the pleasure of avoiding these stock standard insults.

If you're a stay-at-home mum, I'm sorry but you're lazy, and everyone hates you, especially working mums. Because apparently you do nothing all day, because mothers with full-time jobs can keep their kids happy, healthy, and functioning, all whilst working full time. They're doing exactly what you're doing but also having this little thing on the side called a full-time job. They can "do it all," so why can't you? Because of course you can work full time outside of your home and watch kids at exactly the same time. Working mothers manage to work and look after their kids without any sort of child care because, as you know, they do it *all* without any help from anyone, so why can't you? Just attach some bionic limbs, you lazy stay-at-home mothers.

Working mums, sorry, everybody hates you too. You selfishly choose work over your children. You should be charging into primary school every lunchtime so that your ten year old can suckle at your teat. Clearly you are a child-hating, man-hating destroyer of society. You should be getting pleasure from being a "real" woman and doing woman's work. You and your fancy notions of working are an affront to our society. What next? You'll want to learn to read? Or vote? You are a burden on society because you working means we need far too much child care, and you have contributed to the destruction of traditional family values. Because of you, housing prices have skyrocketed. The very fabric of society has been destroyed because you wanted to do something outside of the home. Who wants to ever do anything aside from being with their kids? Who do you think you are? A man! Why not put on devil horns and be done with it?

Do you work from home and have flexible hours like me? You smug fucker, I bet you thought you had the perfect balance. Well, you're the most hated of the lot. You're not a real stay-at-home mum because you actually want to get paid work done at times, and you're not a real working mum because seriously you just sit in pj's until noon. You work too much to be able to properly look after your children, but you don't work enough to be a Wonder Woman. Some women have it all; you have nothing. You're bitches. You shouldn't even be allowed to have children. You don't even take your lives seriously enough to choose to be a "real" working mother or a "real" stay-at-home mother. How can you even parent?

Do you breastfeed? I breastfed my daughter for eighteen months and the twins for five months, so I know your kind. I know all of your games. You are a stuck-up bitch who lords your mammary glands over everyone else. You only breastfeed because you want to show other women that you're better than them. In fact, you probably wouldn't care if your baby starved. You depraved nipple-possessing heathen. You are just using breastfeeding as an excuse to show off your hooties. Stop ripping off your top in the middle of shopping centres, screaming, "Behold my glorious bosom, givers of life, the ultimate super food," then doinking several people on their heads before commencing feeding. We know you have boobs—we get it—but we don't want to see them unless they're in something sexy and being used to elicit the pleasure of the male gaze. So please, just put those norks away unless you're being seductive with them. Then it is, of course, hunky dory.

Do you formula feed? Wow, why did you even have children? You must hate them. You don't want to breastfeed so much that your bitter little nip nips won't even express a drop of precious golden milk just as God intended. Why don't you just feed your child heroine because that's what formula is!?! Stop acting like it is some sort of scientifically created nourishment that will help you feed your hungry child. It's toxic garbage. I mean, my goodness, what are you thinking, giving your child one of the most highly tested and highly studied products of all time? Don't you know that formula-fed babies are dumber than breastfed babies? They're going to end up being unemployable. Thanks for bringing another burden into the world.

Do you mix feed? What the hell is wrong with you? Are you pro-feeding or something? You just care that a child is happy, healthy, and fed? Pick a side, you freak! You're as bad as mothers who work from home with flexible hours. You're not enough of anything. For shame. If you can't decide how to feed your child, then how are you going to decide on anything else? Do you even parent, brah?

Do you make updates about how proud you are of your children? Well, stop. Nobody wants to read about the good things in your life. In fact, you must only be writing good things because you are a closet child hater. You're covering your arse. What a beeyotch. I cannot believe you are so twisted that you think your friends would actually want to take joy in the things that make you happy. As if friends care about your happiness. Next, you'll be telling me about how happy you are with your exercise regime. As if I take joy in your joy. Taking joy in other people's achievements is weird. We must all be miserable and bitter. Kill all the tall poppies.

Do you post updates asking questions or asking for support during difficult times? If you were a good mum, you would already know all the answers. You're just a drama queen looking for people to give you sympathy. How dare you want sympathy on a hard day? How dare you expect your friends to love and support you? You're a mother; you don't deserve love and respect and support anymore. Seriously, everyone is sick of hearing your whinging. Why don't you just post about the good times and save us all the troubles of hearing your woes? You're such a fucking downer.

Do you exercise? Yes? Well, isn't that nice for you? Your children must be running the streets injecting hemp oil into their eyeballs whilst you do that. There is no possible way for you to do that if you are looking after your children properly. You can't do it in your lounge room whilst they nap. You can't get a babysitter. You can't possibly get their other parent to look after them. You must simply be neglecting them for your vanity. If you loved your children, you would be spending time with them, not taking thirty minutes a day to exercise. How can you even think of taking thirty minutes a day for yourself? There is no "yourself" in FAMILY!

Do you exercise? No? Ewwww. You are an embarrassment to your children. Not only that, but you are a terrible influence on them. Your disgustingly unhealthy lifestyle is rubbing off on your kids. They are going to become sedentary and just sit watching TV all day. Because that's what you do; if you're not exercising, you must be just sitting on your butt doing nothing. If you loved your children, you would be exercising and demonstrating a positive lifestyle to them. You're all going to become morbidly obese. There is no other option. There is no middle ground. Stop the madness.

Are you a single mum? You've ruined your children's lives because you haven't provided them with a stable home, because a stable home isn't about love and support—it's about how many parents are in the house. Who cares that you go above and beyond to ensure that your children are supported and nurtured? It's all about numbers.

Are you part of a couple or married? You intolerant, fake human being. Your smugness sickens us all. Your kids will be jerks because you think you're better than everyone else because you have a traditional home life. Well, you don't. Your kids will actually be less creative and smart because you haven't provided them with enough diversity.

Are you a lesbian mum? (See above: *Are you a single mum?)* On top of that, you and your wanton ways will be the ruin of our society, the ruin. Just like those working mothers. Your children will all come out hating men because we all know that lesbian equals man-hater. So they'll all become lesbians. Including the boys. They'll be lesbian boys. Oh, and you're ruining religion. What would Jesus do? Apparently go and harass lesbians online and threaten them. He'll hang out with thieves, prostitutes, and tax collectors but apparently when it comes to homosexuality, he suddenly wants to start trolling for trouble?

Are you a feminist mum? First off, you're ugly, and hairy, and also a man-hater. You shouldn't be allowed to have sons because you hate males. Your daughters will come out being wilful bitches, otherwise known as being like your average man. They won't want to squeeze babies out of their vagingo because feminists despise children and anything to do with men, like sperm, and so our whole population will be decimated. Thanks for bringing about the destruction of the human race with your silly ideas about equality.

Did you have a vaginal birth? Ewww. Your sons will hate vag now and be gay, and apparently there's something wrong with that. Your daughter will love it so will be a lesbian, and apparently there's something wrong with that too. Same with breastfeeding. Just don't do it.

Did you have a C-section? Wow, too posh to push. I don't care about your health conditions and how you and your baby/babies could die, or you could be permanently incontinent. You posh bitch.

And now for my favourite round of shaming, courtesy of a Facebook chain post on Mother's Day, 2015.

Did you keep your child in your belly for long enough? Here's the status update that was chaining its way around.

In honour of Mother's Day, post the name, birthday, due date, and weight of your child(ren). Then post in comments so your fellow mothers can post onto their wall.

Name:

Birthday:

Due Date:

Weight:

If you are before your due date, in particular if you are more than three weeks beforehand (37 weeks is full term, so you are still okay and your fanwah is functional from 37-39 weeks—not perfect, just okay; don't get too proud of your nethers), you have a sucky vagina. If you are late with big babies, you're a lazy chocolate-eating beast who poisoned your child in the womb. If you had it on the due date, you're anal. Good luck with that.

So just let it be known, whatever kind of mamma you are, you suck. For the record, I had my daughter vaginally at 35 weeks, I breastfed her for 18 months—she was a bottle refuser—and I returned to work part time when she was 18 months. I had my twins at 32 weeks via emergency C-section, breastfed them for 5 months, then switched to formula, and began working from home as a writer. As you can see, I suck on multiple levels. If you too suck, don't worry. We can suck together. Let's bring it in for a virtual hug. Mmmmmmmmm, that was nice. We can be part of each other's girl tribe.

Invisible Prejudices

When you get out of the nuthouse, everyone feels more comfortable talking about their own struggles with you. They figure that you're so screwed up that you can't possibly judge them, and let's face it: it's kind of true. I actually mostly enjoy that aspect because it means that people feel comfortable talking to me. Even total strangers seem to feel as if I'm a safe space for them. But unfortunately, it leads to some people saying hurtful stuff to you without them even realising it. You really need your tribe of madwomen to talk to when these things happen because nobody else understands quite the way they do. There is one incident that happened fairly soon after I left the madhouse that clearly reveals people's supposedly "invisible" prejudices around the notion of mental illness and, even more so, being in a psychiatric hospital.

A few months after getting out of hospital, one of my friends told me for the umpteenth time that, *at this rate, she was going to need to be admitted into an institution if her family didn't pull their finger out*. She's not the only one who said this to me upon my exit. She was just the main "offender." People still say this to me because I'm supposed to understand that it is the pinnacle of bad things that can happen. They assume that because I was in a psychiatric hospital, I'll automatically understand that getting intensive, professional support marks just how fucked up your world is, and nothing could be worse. It's kind of hurtful for people to imply that your life is their idea of a worst-case scenario. Now I understand that a lot of people reading this will think, "So the fuck what? Isn't going into a mental home the worst thing that could happen? Isn't everyone in there really crazy and fucked up?" Ummmm, not exactly, and don't be mean. In reality, because I have been in a psychiatric hospital, I know darned well that there are far worse things than going in hospital. Namely, denying that you are mentally ill and forcing your loved ones to live through your paranoia and rages untreated. Self-medicating with drugs and alcohol, putting your family into debt, running away, or committing suicide, thus leaving your children with abandonment issues, and oh so many other things are far worse than getting intensive treatment.

As for the crazy and fucked up, a standard psychiatric hospital and a hospital for the criminally insane are two very different things. You don't slap a bunch of women with PND or cops with PTSD in with paedophiles and serial killers. It's just not even close to the same thing. And that's the problem. People subconsciously lump us all together. Hidden deep down, there is this thought that everyone under the *mental illness* umbrella are all disturbed individuals, totally disconnected with reality. If you question someone on their beliefs, they'll no doubt say that they see depression and extreme psychosis as two very different things. But despite their words to the contrary, they'll still treat people with depression and anxiety like they don't know what is happening and can't really be trusted.

This same friend also freaked out when someone she knew suggested she had PND. She complained bitterly about how she was going to go to the doctor to take a test to prove them wrong. And can I just say, nothing says mentally tip top like running into your doctor's office and screaming, *I'M NOT CRAZY!* It was as if the notion was so abhorrent that she needed to rush off to prove otherwise immediately. PND was a stigma she couldn't accept because people would think she was a bad mother. BAM, there you have it. Invisible prejudice now visible. Societal norms dictate that people with depression are not capable people. And people who seek intensive help for it are cowards and should just soldier on... poisoning everything they touch. Treatment is for the weak; anger and resentment is for the strong. People in our liberated time say how they can't believe how patients, even as late as the 1970s, were subjected to horrific treatments. These supposedly beneficial treatments for the mentally ill included such things as rotation therapy, which was like being put on the spinning swings at a carnival but for hours, not minutes; immersion therapy, where patients were kept submerged for not just hours but sometimes days in water; and radiation therapy, where patients were exposed to things like radium. Inhumane treatments that would drive any sane person into the depths of despair. Patients were often kept sedated so that they weren't a bother to staff.

To be honest, I am beginning to realise we really haven't come that far, as society would like to sedate mental illness from its consciousness. Sure, it's okay for the odd celebrity or journalist to have depression, as long as they stick to portraying the stereotype of it, but only bring that nasty crap near us once you're better and productive again. Please, don't tell us about your reoccurring battles, and certainly don't thrust it into our faces with suicide. People want to avoid it because it makes them uncomfortable, because they view it as being the worst thing ever. Heck, even in my own life, people balk at the idea of me being mentally ill. They try to gloss over it because they cannot reconcile the fact that I seem to be funny, smart, articulate, a great mother, and not entirely unfortunate looking, and yet somehow I suffer from depression and anxiety. "Oh, you're so hilarious, you're not really depressed. You're a super woman. You're just exhausted." Well, I'm going to have to burst their bubble. I'm all those good things, but I am also depressed. Not just a little blue, not in a tizzy, but chronically and clinically depressed.

I went to a novel-pitching event in 2014; other participants thought I was confident and a bit glamorous, and some thought I was a mindless, pretty bimbo. I know this because one person was actually rude enough to ask me if I was there to sell my manuscript or my body. It cut me deeply that I had gone to all that effort to appear professional and had been insulted by a fellow pitcher. They saw a strong, confident woman that they wanted to cut down. Someone they wanted to fail so that they could succeed. They didn't realise it wasn't a bit of a mask that I was wearing like they were, but a carefully constructed performance that I have for public rituals. Because I know damn well what a burden people find me if I let all of me out to play. That the nervous, shy girl, who threw up before entering, would not be considered good company. So I only show parts of me, and I'm not even sure they're the best parts of me, but they are the socially acceptable parts of me. Humour, grooming, smiles, the odd profound insight (but not too many) and self-deprecation. Heck, the day before going, I was lamenting to a friend, who was also pitching, that I was worried that the not-so-acceptable bits of me would slip out. Bits that are so objectionable by our invisible prejudice. Surprisingly, she told me that my awkward interjections at random moments were what made me loveable, and she kind of thought they were my "shtick." I'm as Celtic as they come, so I don't think I can have a "shtick," but it was comforting to know if I didn't manage to keep myself on lockdown, then it wouldn't be all bad.

I don't write this to shame anyone who has lamented to me how they might end up in the nuthouse and just how fucked up it would be to go to the same place I went. *Gee, thanks for letting me know what a loser you think I am.* Or to shame the person who was so rude to me to try to cut me down at a pitching event. Although she should feel a little ashamed. I write it more to get people thinking and to start a conversation about the way people really view mental illness rather than the PC things they think they're supposed to. We cannot start actually addressing people's true feelings about mental health if we're in denial about them. People often can say they're okay about mental health and that they're totally understanding about all the issues, but if someone said to them that they might have depression, their reaction is often akin to being accused of being a racist.

Part of the reason that I hate these stereotypes and bias so much is because I personally know just how damaging they can be. The first time I was diagnosed with postnatal depression was nine months after my beautiful daughter was born. I couldn't have been more in love with her. I thought she was the most beautiful thing I had ever seen. Every tear shredded my heart, and I wanted nothing more than to protect her. Sure, I was exhausted; she had reflux, which wasn't diagnosed until late, so she was incredibly unsettled—nobody gets sleep with a baby that has genuine reflux. And on top of that, she was also diagnosed with hip dysplasia late and so ended up in a spica cast from armpit to ankle, with two rounds of surgery, which was very uncomfortable for her, and very distressing for us to see her in so much pain. Both conditions I had been asking my GP about for months, only to be dismissed. At four months, I switched GPs and am so glad that I did. Always listen to your intuition.

I had a baby in a cast from ankle to armpit and severe reflux at the same time. It wasn't easy. I was exhausted, I was teary, and I was suicidal. But hey, I loved my baby, and this was a trying circumstance—how could I possibly have postnatal depression? Women with postnatal depression all hate their babies, right? They think they smell weird and will not hold them? Wrong. Sure, there are some women who fit into that perfect stereotypical box, but many women do not. Only knowing the stereotypes and not the facts meant that I delayed seeking help because I didn't think for a moment that I could have postnatal depression. Some people think perpetuating this stereotype helps raise awareness, but it really doesn't when it can be misleading.

Many women are *depressed* postnatally, not utterly disconnected or psychotic. They love their kids; they just have zero resilience left. They put that beautiful baby to bed and then lie on the kitchen floor, sobbing uncontrollably until the baby wakes again, or they vomit. They can't sleep for fear something will happen to their baby. They can't unwind because everything they do, they are sure it is somehow wrong and ruining that little baby's life. That baby that they love more than anything. Essentially, it is exactly the same as the fears all mothers have but times that by ten and never ever switch it off, not even for a cup of tea. Women with PND are just like every other mother, just more so. We're not scary, we don't need to feel ashamed, and we need compassion and support. And even if you previously thought you couldn't understand us, you really can because we're just like you.

The medical profession has recently separated Postnatal Depression into two categories: Postnatal Depression and Postnatal Psychosis. The latter deals with those more extreme cases, such as the rejection of the baby upfront, all the way up to those murder-suicide cases that break everyone's hearts. I have a theory that in years to come, it will be split again to add a third category, postnatal *anxiety*. (Even as I write this memoir it is becoming in vogue for people to start using the term postnatal anxiety, looks like I was right.) Because I think that gives a more understandable definition. Mothers are anxious creatures to begin with; we women with PND just tend to excel at it. High fives all around. We won at something... even though it's nail biting, stomach churning, and hair pulling.... But a win is a win, right? And adding this term might help more women to come forward because it doesn't have the stereotype of baby hating and disconnection attached to it. Just a thought.

The Charlotte Dawson Effect

For the person with high anxiety or depression, even something as common as using social media is a death trap waiting to happen. As I sit sipping my morning cup of tea, I appear every bit normal and relaxed. Nobody would know the inner turmoil that I feel when getting into cyber altercations with trolls. And to be honest, I'm always so quick with a joke that most people wouldn't know how upset I get during cyber-attacks. They might guess I'm a bit pissed off, but they don't realise that internally, I'm curled up in the foetal position sucking on my blanky. But unfortunately, I have been known to have what I term "Charlotte Dawson" moments. Trust me, they are nowhere near as thrilling as my "Oprah" moments. I think it's probably pertinent that I have a bit of a rant about cyber "trolls" and why it is so hard for those of us with depression to move on.

But before I do that, let me quickly address one important issue concerning metalanguage… because I don't want people to get upset and complain about me "troll shaming" because I'm not. I love good-luck trolls. Not only do I appreciate the ever so cute good-luck troll but the rest of trollkind too. I understand the value of them guarding forbidden bridges, and I agree that goats can be quite delicious. And I'm sure that genuine cyber trolls are actually really upset about arsehole humans being called trolls, as they probably guard super-secret electronic highways. I am positive that they are out there protecting us from seeing things that are so extraordinary that they would literally blow our tiny minds, resulting in brains being splattered onto computer screens globally. We don't want that.

So perhaps I shouldn't further defame the noble troll and actually refer to these people as what they are... nasty pasties? Bitches? Shrivelled-up bitter souls with nothing better to do than tear others down? Dickheads? We really need to come up with a better name than "troll" for them. I feel the need to use quotation marks for "trolls" from now on to differentiate them from actual trolls who, I have already said, provide valuable bridge-guarding services. Honestly, how trolls had their reputation so maligned that they've gone from being loner types who guard bridges and enjoy snacking on Bovidae loins to being a bunch of people who actively seek you out and just keep on hounding you is beyond me. On behalf of humanity, I apologise to the noble troll for my use of the word "troll." I sincerely hope society comes up with a better word soon so that you can guard your bridges in peace. I do understand that the term came from people "tolling/patrolling for trouble," but trolls seem to be the ones coping the flak from it, rather than patrollers. I'm a fantasy lover so very protective of my real trolls.

Actually, stuff society. I shall come up with a better name. Bear with me for a moment whilst I share a story with you. A while back, I walked my angels around the park and saw a woman sitting innocently eating some hot chips, or French Fries, as our friends across the pond call them. Sure enough, it wasn't long before a gang of seagulls started heavying her for some of those salty sticks of goodness. Welcome to Australia. First, a few squawked their beaks off, and then they were joined by more until the poor woman was being practically deafened. Soon after, things turned ugly. The seagulls were no longer happy to sit back and catcall, so they launched an offensive. They wanted those tasty chips, they needed those chips, and they were going to take those chips by force if necessary. The woman soon packed up her stuff and moved somewhere else. The same thing happened. So she moved again but dumped a few chips first. The seagulls ate the chips, then set chase. This continued until the woman finally left the park. It didn't matter how many chips she gave them, and it didn't matter how many times she moved; the seagulls kept coming until she had fled. Seagulls like chips. Who can blame them? Chips are delicious. Same with "trolls" or should I say "cyber seagulls." Once they see a delicious hot morsel, they must have it. It isn't the chip's fault that it is delicious. The chip hasn't done anything wrong by being delicious. It simply is a delicious thing. Just like it isn't a "cyber chip's" fault that the "cyber seagull" seeks to devour it. Seagulls are loud aggressive things that eat chips for breakfast. That's just their nature.

"Cyber seagulls," like real seagulls, have very little capacity to respect boundaries. If you block them, they will simply try to get your attention through friends' accounts or follow you to a different platform. You see, the "cyber seagull" has some deep issues. They believe that not only are they important in their own world but they must be important in yours. So when you block these self-important folk, they go completely troppo. They'll start complaining about things like free speech. You can explain that you're not a government organisation so you blocking them doesn't actually impact on Freedom of Speech even one little bit, but they won't care. I still recommend blocking them despite the fact that they will go feral on your arse; it's just that you may need to do so repeatedly to several accounts and across multiple platforms. Because the "cyber seagull" will hound you for quite some time, just like the real deal. You are a tasty chip, and they must eat you.

For some reason, they need perfect strangers to put up with their issues. The idea that someone that they have never met cuts them out of their life really bothers them. Yes, it's sad for them to live like that, but it isn't our responsibility to put up with it while thinking we're helping. It is their responsibility to stop, think about their priorities, and then seek help. Being a cyber punching bag for someone does not help them, and it destroys you. We need to construct our lives and our cyber lives so that it brings us as much joy and strength as possible. This is particularly important if you have depression or anxiety. You simply don't have the resilience to endure constant abuse for no reason. And nobody should have to put up with that. Put your energy into feeding the hungry rather than coping with abuse. If we have seagulls in our life draining our energy, then we need to remove them; otherwise, they will keep deafening us with the wail of their own needs and totally consume our own. There are trained professionals who are strong enough to withstand the noise. Those with sensitive hearing don't need to feel responsible to do so. Simply put on your earmuffs and move on.

Now there's an image: a hot chip strutting around with earmuffs on whilst seagulls scream nearby. I guess what I'm trying to say is that if you're being "trolled," it's probably because you're awesome. You've brought attention to yourself by being funny, or sweet, or wise, and these people just can't stand for others to have that attention, so they descend. So don't feel bad that you're being attacked. You're amazing; you're a hot chip. Don't change who you are because of arseholes, but don't feel the need to subject yourself to it either. Just, ya know, ignore it. Easier said than done, right?

In 2014, Charlotte Dawson, a famous Australian/New Zealander former model and television personality, committed suicide after tweeting to the twitter cyber seagulls that they had won. There was a huge outcry. People said things ranging from, "stupid bitch should have ignored them," to, "those bullies have blood on their hands." It, of course, can't be that simple. At least in my expert (Note: I am an expert of nothing at all) opinion, it can't be that simple. My own experiences over the last few years have really helped open my eyes. I've been cyber spanked previously, and I wasn't confident enough in myself to be able to step back and think about it. I allowed it to fill me with anxiety to the point where I became physically ill. But thankfully after my time in the Mother and Baby unit, I am now able to be much more reflective and deal with these circumstances.

I, like many modern mothers, was once part of an online parenting group. Generally, we shared cute stories and pics and asked for advice. As is true of all social interactions, you click with some people, and you clash with others. I naturally found myself migrating towards the misfits, the clowns, the geeks. Otherwise known as the beautifully flawed. You can always recognise a kindred weirdo. (Thanks for reading and laughing along, much appreciated.) There really are few greater joys than finding a fellow freak. Us dorks tend to band together and don't really like to be told what to do, and we stand up for other people being put down. We've been shunned our whole life and know how it feels to be on the outside. But being that we are a bit different, our defence of other vulnerable people is also different. When people start getting tense and telling people what products they *must* use or how they *must* interact with their baby or what they *must* feed their children or any other *must*, I tend to crack a joke to lighten the mood. For most people, it works. My fellow jokers are attracted to the humour like a clown moth to a novelty flame, and soon we're all having a good giggle, and the crisis is averted. Unfortunately, that doesn't always work.

Sure, the merry band of misfits let out a collective sigh of relief, and most other people think, thank goodness for the distraction, but unfortunately, this levity only serves to highlight the darkness in some people's souls. They want control, they crave control, and my joke has robbed them of that. So what do they do? They lash out, they twist the joke, they pretend it is a personal attack, and they raise an army of followers and have them make specific, directed attacks. Like, seriously, I made a joke about a pleather skirt that I own, and how I shouldn't have made a major purchase whilst in the nuthouse, and a woman in a Facebook parenting group managed to convince people that I was making a joke about her new leather couch. Like I was supposed to know she had a new couch, let alone what it was made of. How the fuck does a person get me attacking their couch out of me talking about my own fashion failure? *Sorry, pleather skirt. I still think you rock; no matter what the others say, you're no failure.* So random joke about random a thing gets met with specific, personal attacks. Not exactly a fair reaction. Unfortunately, when you're depressed, any attack, no matter how unfounded, turns your stomach. Anxiety starts to get out of control, and your urge to smooth things over becomes overwhelming. So what do I do? Try to make more jokes and try to make people smile. Further illuminating the gaping chasm these angry people have in their worldview, which results in more nasty, personal attacks. I continue to make random jokes about things, not people (unless said people are my fellow misfits and they love it), yet they continue to escalate with vitriol.

With Charlotte Dawson, her tactic, when confronted with cyber seagulls, seemed to be to try to build awareness and educate. I have never met the woman, but she seemed to be rather earnest and actually pleading with people. I do understand her role on television was to criticise, but she seemed to be quite different from her television personality on her personal Twitter account. She didn't fall back on humour—that's my crutch—she fell back on trying to illuminate. Regardless of the defence mechanism, her attempts similarly failed and only reflected the darkness within the attackers. It didn't change them; it made the people angrier because they had it in their mind that they must have power, and they must have control. Charlotte Dawson and I have wasted our time. I can see that now. Some people are so hell-bent on proving their self-worth to themselves that they have no time for anything different. They will lash out and tear down those who are silly enough to attempt to use any coping methods like humour or education. They need to fuel their own needs by destroying all others. Yes, they're tragic; yes, they need help. But only they can do that. Only they can change themselves. Trying to smooth things over, trying to enlighten them, just gives them fodder. They need help, but it is their responsibility to seek it, not ours.

What have I learned from this? That I am no more capable of *not* trying to make people smile with humour than Charlotte Dawson was of *not* trying to educate others. I am still vulnerable, and the attacks make me feel sick. It doesn't matter that I know I'm a good person and that my friends know it, too; I'm still able to be shaken. So what do I do about it? I block cyber seagulls and quickly. I don't need to interact with people just "seagulling" for trouble. I have learned the lesson of what I term the *Charlotte Dawson Effect*, and I have moved on. I know I can't stop trying to make people happy by making jokes, and that my humour pains the cyber seagulls because it means they begin to lose the control they are white-knuckling to maintain. For me, the solution is simple: no contact. Does it work? Pretty much. People still occasionally hound me. I guess the fact that people take time out of their day to post on my clownish ways really is an honour... but seeing their abuse of me doesn't enrich my life in any way. In fact, blocking these abusive people gives me the freedom to be me. I can joke and have fun. I can comment freely and be myself and not have to censor myself because the people who will try to twist it can no longer see me, and I can't see them hurting me by trying to turn my bringing laughter and joy to others into a hideous sin.

And now for my hot tip to the fellow anxious individual on social media: construct your reality in a way that strengthens you. Make sure you talk to your tribe if things are getting on top of you. Keep those who make you feel good and strive to be a better person close to you. Remove those who try to make your soul as black as theirs. Don't change who you are. You are the best you that you can be. Don't give your time away to bad situations. Be you! Be you in all your glory. Let people love you for who you are, and don't lessen yourself for fear of others. As the old saying goes, you could be the juiciest peach in the world, but there will always be someone out there who hates peaches. The peach is fine, the peach is perfect, there is nothing wrong with the peach, the peach doesn't have to change, and the peach doesn't have to change people's minds to think it is delicious. Be the peach.

Not only does cyber space suck for the highly anxious or depressive types, but so does the news. I'm not even talking about the comment sections on news articles. For the love of chocolate, don't read the comment section, but the actual news itself can be mega bleak. I periodically have to ban myself from watching the news because I can become so upset that I can no longer function. Some people think that this is terrible. That you mustn't bury your head in the sand because nothing changes if good people do nothing. Which is of course true, but there are limits.

Don't get me wrong—call bullshit where you see it. Slavery didn't end because everyone quietly minded their own business, women didn't get the vote by speaking sweetly, and apartheid didn't end because people followed societal expectations. Don't let people try to shame you into silence by calling you a do-gooder or saying you should mind your own business. Where would we be if Steve Biko sat on his hands because people told him to stop? It's easy to stand with the crowd. It takes courage to stand alone.

People called the likes of Gandhi and Mandela do-gooders, lawbreakers, holier than thou, wanting more than they should, arrogant, overreactors, inhumane people wanting to upset others, and all sorts of other names. People tried to shame and threaten and beat them into silence. Thankfully, they showed staggering courage and tenacity and stood outside the crowds of their time and stood up for what is right. Both were imprisoned, both suffered hideous treatment, and Gandhi was even assassinated for his efforts, yet their legacies live on. Their changes made all of our lives better. Not just people in South Africa and India, but the vibrations of their influence were felt across the globe. Because ending persecution and bigotry anywhere helps everyone everywhere. How many people like them do we deride today when we should be supporting them?

Gandhi once said something akin to "happiness is when your actions and ideas are in harmony." I'd like a slice of that happiness. The happiness of living to your own moral code. That's actually my aim this year: to be me and to be happy about it. To get brutally serious for a moment, every day, we make judgements, and it's important to do so. I judge paedophilia as wrong, I judge child abuse as wrong, I judge domestic violence as wrong, I judge hate crimes as wrong. I judge the beginnings of these things as wrong—sexism, racism, homophobia, ableism, and so on. My aim for this year is to stand firm in my own moral judgements, to speak up about them, support those who likewise speak out, and not to be shamed into silence by those who would prefer bigotry to go unquestioned. We all make our own judgements; it's time we owned them.

I know that taking a stand is important. I know that being informed is important. But sometimes, I just have to say, "Fuck this shit. I'm going on a news ban." I was actually on a news ban just last month, or I honestly would have been too terrified to leave the house. I'd already found myself limiting my movements because I was so anxious about the world we live in and how cruel it can be. Two percent of the people on this planet are despicable human beings, and at times, I cannot hear another thing about them and the horrors they inflict on others, or I will just curl up into a ball and cry until I vomit. I can't do that. I have three kids—people tell me I have a husband too—and I obviously have to put out gripping books such as this one. And sometimes after reading the news, I feel as if I need to bleach my brain and take a rest. So that's exactly what I do. And then, when I'm ready, I get back into it. I'm no use to anyone if I'm a jibbering mess. Sometimes you have to take care of yourself first, and then, once you're strong enough, go back to advocating for others. I don't mean being aggressive and self-centred in a nasty way. I simply mean that it's okay to step back every now and then. It's okay to be kind to yourself.

Treat Yourself like a Friend

Sometimes I think we're much nicer to our friends than we are to ourselves. At times, what we really need to do is step back and think, *What would I say if this was happening to a friend?* I bet our words would be infinitely kinder if they were to a friend than what we would say to ourselves. A while back, I wrote a letter to an acquaintance who was going through a tough time. Upon reading it, I thought to myself, "Wow, I wish someone would say something like this to me," and then I realised, "Hey, I should really be saying this kind of stuff to me." So I'm going to write a letter to myself right now. It's kind of like those *20 Tips You'd Give Your 16 Year Old Self* things, except it's for right now.

Dear Robin,

I know it was only this morning that we chatted, in the shower when we constructed the best comeback ever to people who give unsolicited parenting advice, but I thought I'd pop back now to have a few more words.

Firstly, you're not hideous, so stop avoiding looking in mirrors. No, seriously, look in the mirror long enough every single day to wash your face and put moisturiser on. It's really not that bad. You even have a friend who thinks that you look like you're wearing makeup all the time. She's a nutritionist, so she knows what healthy skin looks like. Stop avoiding the mirror. Full props that you've come so far that you no longer cover your mirrors so that you don't accidentally have to see yourself—that's progress, but it's time to take it further. The mirror is not haunted, a demon is not going to pop out, you are not a demon, and your face is not hideous; look in the mirror every day. You can do it. You look fine. Your daughter thinks you're beautiful, so unless you want to call her a filthy little liar, you better start believing it.

Secondly, that conversation went fine. Whatever conversation you just had and enjoyed in the moment, and are now worrying yourself sick about, was just as enjoyable in the moment for the other person as it was for you. No; really, it was. You neither spoke too much, nor too little. Conversations are fluid and don't have to go on an exact 50/50 ratio. Sometimes you'll speak more, and sometimes other people will speak more; that's life. And guess what? Even if you did say something that unintentionally offended the other person, who cares? How many times have friends said insensitive things to you about depression or dyslexia, and you still like them? How many times have you received unsolicited parenting advice from certain people, and you still hang out with them? Lots. Many lots! Sometimes we all say stupid stuff, sometimes we all say insensitive stuff. We are not robots; we're human beings, and that's why we love each other. We're wacky, we're weird, we sometimes do the most bizarre stuff, and that's what makes us unique. So quite reliving that conversation, it was fine and you're fine.

Thirdly, yes you got frustrated with your kids. No, you're not proud of yourself, but no, you don't need to dwell on it and punish yourself by thinking that you are the worst parent in the world. You didn't hit anyone, you didn't swear at anyone, and you didn't expose anyone to their worst fear in order to punish them. Yep, you raised your voice. No, it's not ideal, but you made reparations, and you don't do it every week. Nobody is perfect—we all lose our cool every now and then. Especially those people in your life who deny that they do. You have seen each and every last one of them lose it worse than you ever have; so give yourself a break. You don't have to hold yourself to such a high standard. Your kids are going to be fine. They're going to be more than fine—they're going to be brilliant—and you don't have to be superhuman in order to do it. And you don't want to set an example of self-flagellation for having occasional slipups. Just make your reparations and reconnections and move on. For the love of Xena, *move on!*

Fourthly, stop thinking about it. You've already done enough overthinking to last yourself a lifetime. You've thought about everything you need to, everything you don't need to, and all the things that no person should ever have to think. Heck, you've thought of everything there ever was to think of except for something truly useful like a cure for cancer. So you're all good. You've done your bit for "overthinking kind." You should be given a gold watch and allowed to retire. In fact, any new issue that comes up, you've already thought of the answer. You're ahead of the game, having gone over it all in your head in minute detail before. It's time for you to retire from overthinking things. You're all thought up. You've thought all of the thoughts and all of the things. You're done now; go have a nap. Naps are fantastic. You deserve one. But not before you read the next point. You need to read it. I need you to read it.

Fifthly, and possibly most importantly, for the love of warrior princesses everywhere, when you go to the cinema, stop letting your husband choose the movie. He has terrible taste in movies. Whenever he chooses the movie, you're both disappointed. Not only do you have to sit through a vaguely traumatic movie that he has promised is a comedy, you then have to hear him complain about it for ages. Whenever you choose the movie, you merely have to hear him whinge about it and undermine your choice in the lead up, but then he raves about how good it was afterwards. It's time to make a stand—everybody has different strengths, and his isn't picking good movies. It's doing chin-ups or the salmon ladder. So no more compromise on the movie front; it just leads to disappointment for everyone. Do you really want to sit through one more movie where the dog dies, or the guy dies in a box? Of course not. You have excellent taste in movies. Just go with your own instincts.

Fond Regards,
Robin

Don't you think it's time that we were as nice to ourselves as we were our friends? Shouldn't we have our own back? After all, we are the person that we will have the longest relationship with in our lives. We're there at the start and we're there at the end. It's high time we started being kind to ourselves.

How about you go and write yourself a letter? A letter to yourself now—sure, it'd be nice to give your younger self some sage advice and words of comfort, but that ship has well and truly sailed. So for today, tell yourself what you need to hear right now. What would you say to you if you were your best friend? Instead of saying, "I'm surrounded by arseholes, so I must suck," correct yourself to, "I'm surrounded by arseholes because I'm so tolerant. I might start setting some boundaries to take care of this issue but not lose my kindness." Put that same positive spin on anything you'd say to yourself that you would to a friend. Lisa M Hayes says, "Be careful what you tell yourself because you're listening."

I think, at the moment, there are a lot of mothers who are hurting. Mothers who didn't get that childhood that demonstrated to them how to deal with intense emotions and tough times. There was a big push to just shut up. If you had big feelings, you were either punished for being a brat or, if you were lucky, someone tried to distract you instead of smacking you. Both of these things can be techniques (full disclosure: I'm not a smacker), but they cannot be the only tools in the toolbox for dealing with kids and emotions because they simply don't teach people how to process their feelings and how to outwardly react appropriately. They simply teach that those emotions are unwelcome, and they need to stop. So then we have kids, and they're crying, or screaming, and we have to work out what to do, and all we've had modelled to us is a smack or being sent away. That makes things challenging because, deep down, we know how scary that can be to be on the receiving end of.

People like to talk big and say, "I got a smack, and it never did me any harm." Usually said in a really aggressive tone, which makes it abundantly clear that some harm has been done because why else are they so angry and defensive? Why can't they discuss it calmly? Probably because they were never taught those skills. Sure, we can all discuss things calmly when things are easy, but doing so under pressure is a real skill and one that is often overlooked when raising kids. When we were kids, our tantrums were inconvenient and shut down swiftly through fear. We learned to shut up when someone bigger and stronger was around. But we actually needed to learn how to communicate, even when in distress, and not to just silently rage and cower in fear.

And to be honest, I don't even believe these people who keep telling me how great the good old days were, when a belting apparently never did anyone any harm. To be frank, the next time someone tells me how good the old days were, and how much better it was, I might remind them that apparently they didn't know that paedophilia was a big deal and didn't have mechanisms in place for dealing with it back in the good old days. A couple of things that keep coming up in the *Australian Royal Commission Into Child Abuse* is that the child victims didn't report because they feared they would get in trouble with adults for causing a problem and that their word would not be believed over an adult's. The adults who received the reports kept saying that back then they didn't know what a big deal it was and that they felt the kids would just get over it. And this response echoed across institutions and religions. The adults indicated that they felt that if they just kept silent and moved on, all would be okay. But it wasn't okay. Multiple suicides have resulted from past generations' inability to deal with abuse. Their refusal to accept children as real people with real feelings and real rights, and the refusal to believe that long-term harm comes from abuse suffered in childhood has caused irreparable damage to some individuals.

So, to be honest, all those things they thought were okay back in the good old days, like getting kids to take on adult responsibility, beating kids, and apparently even sexually abusing kids, actually aren't okay. They were harmful then, and they are still harmful now. I'm not really a fan of the good old days and the old methods of dealing with things because they have been so clearly proven to be harmful. And maybe, just maybe, people should STFU about how much better things used to be because they really weren't as amazing as people pretend they were. Yes, paedophilia still takes place today; yes, child abuse still happens, but thankfully most people no longer pretend that it isn't a big deal. There have been institutional changes across the board to ensure that these kinds of things are not swept under the rug. Educational campaigns have been released to let people know that violence in the home impacts on children and to believe kids when they say that they have been subjected to abuse. Other people can glorify the good old days, when you could treat kids like possessions, but I certainly won't. And I certainly won't pretend brutalising your children makes you a better parent.

Furthermore, this fiercely defended nostalgia of the good old days, when a "naughty" kid just needed their "backside warmed up" with a "tap," isn't helpful for mothers of today. We keep getting told how great these times were and how much better kids used to be and how we should be parenting that way and that we're spoiling our kids if we don't. It's mind-boggling the onslaught of criticism we now receive. It is no wonder estimates of postnatal depression are so high. We can't even get supported when all we want to do is love our kids. And we often don't have a model to look back on in order to know how to react firmly but compassionately when our kids are experiencing those big emotions that result in toddler tantrums.

Now I understand that it was a different time, and people claim they didn't know any better. But when you know better, you're supposed to do better, not fiercely defend the old ways. Some more support, so that we can all navigate our way through processing our feelings and communicating effectively, even when under pressure, would solve so many issues. It has far-reaching consequences beyond Postnatal Depression. It is important for tackling domestic violence, alcohol addiction, and so many other big problems our society faces. But unfortunately, we have a large percentage of our population burying their heads in the sand. And that makes me sad.

I'm an Arsehole Parent

The other day my daughter asked me for Smarties for breakfast. Let's be honest: we've all been there; we've all felt like eating chocolate for breakfast. I said no. I told her that they weren't a breakfast food and made her have cereal and toast instead. She was unimpressed. I then shipped her off to preschool, returned home, and ate Smarties for breakfast. Talk about being an arsehole. A hypocritical arsehole at that.

I frequently find myself pulling such arsehole parent moves. Like when my kids want burgers and chips. I don't just buy them from a takeaway shop, but I actually make them. I even have a chip cutter so that the potatoes slices are all even. I parboil them and then pop them in the oven. My husband and my sons claim that they love them. My daughter asks me why I must ruin chips. I can't answer that question. Why I feel the need to do this to her instead of just getting oven fries or McDonald's is beyond me. It's like a sick game where I try to make her like my chips by going to increasingly greater efforts in my preparation, and she becomes increasingly unimpressed.

In fact, the last time I made up my homemade burger and chips, she simply sighed and said, "All things considered, I'd prefer to just have bread and water." You have to hand it to four year olds—they're brutally honest.

I have to admit that even these minor issues make my stomach churn. I question myself on if I should just give her the McDonald's option and not give the "healthy" option. It's a burger and chips; it's going to be unhealthy, no matter what. And then I feel guilty that I might have given her a junk-food addiction. And then I feel guilty about calling it "junk" food and setting up an unhealthy relationship with food. I have ruined her whole life because everything in moderation is fine, and I shouldn't demonise food. And then I start to question my motives. Do I really just want to give in and get takeaway because I'm too lazy to cook? Am I a bad mum who doesn't want to put in the effort? Is the excess fat poisoning her mind and turning her into a discipline problem? Are my kids skinny because I don't treat them enough? And it goes on and on and on. So something as simple as a rejected dinner can become an epic battle in my mind between fear and reality.

Kids reject food. Kids tell you that your armpits smell. Kids tell you that you're ugly, and they want to go live with their ballet teacher. Kids tell you all sorts of things. It's not necessarily a reflection on your quality as a parent. Sure, you might have stinky armpits, but that doesn't make you a bad parent. And hey, maybe their ballet teacher is better looking than you and far more smiley and graceful, but that makes you a jealous parent, not a bad one. And sometimes your kid might just want peanut butter on a spoon; again, that doesn't make you a bad parent. But when anxiety rears its ugly head, it's hard to shake off these negative feelings. Having anxiety is kind of like being "normal" but without the ability to shake things off as quickly. You worry about all the same things that other people do, but then you continue to worry. Then you question yourself, your integrity, and your very soul, until you are rolled up into a little ball and howling. Suffering from anxiety is just like normal life but more so. It's amplified normal. It's super normal. I'm pretty sure what I'm saying is that having anxiety makes you a superhero. Yeah. That's it. That's the point I'm making. We're all fucking heroes.

Although some people think anxiety doesn't make us so much heroic as criminally insane. Every time there is a case of a mother murdering her child, people automatically leap to diagnose that person with postnatal depression. Murdering an innocent victim that is utterly dependent on you isn't exactly heroic. This year (2016), in Australia, there have been several high-profile maternal infanticide cases.

The Australian nation held its collective breath when Sofina Nikat, mother of fourteen-month-old Sanaya, said that her daughter had been stolen by a "black man" whilst they went for their morning walk in Heidelberg West. Nikat claimed the man smelled strongly of alcohol, wore no shoes, was African, between 20-30 years old, and that he pushed her down and then unstrapped little Sanaya from her pram before running off with the toddler.

The story seemed far-fetched. Internet sleuths quickly pointed out the flaws in her story: how could she know the age or gender or ethnicity if she didn't really see them?—how did he unstrap the baby in time?—and what the F does African look like? The continent of Africa contains many countries and ethnicities, so simply "African" doesn't cut it. This isn't 1920s America where a vague story about a "black man" is enough to get everyone gathering their pitchforks. This is Australia. Their suspicions correct, Nikat fairly quickly confessed. A fabled "black man" did not take her baby. She murdered her baby.

Of course this cued the cries of, "She must have had PND" from people on social media. People insisted that the mother be shown compassion because nobody in their right mind would do something so horrible; she must have had postnatal depression. Compassion is an admirable state, but I'll just give you a moment to think about the full statement and let that sink in. People didn't say, "She must have had a psychotic break." They said, "She must have had PND. Nobody in their right mind would do something so horrible, so she must have had postnatal depression." They're basically saying that people with postnatal depression are incapable of reason. This simply isn't true.

There are 25-27 cases of children being murdered by their parents each year in Australia. There are far more cases of PND a year than 27. The gender of the parent responsible for the crime is spread out fairly evenly amongst the genders. So how about social media sleuths and the media stop automatically labelling children murdered by their mother as being a result of PND? The approach is far too simplistic and does not fit the facts.

If it were as simple as it being because of PND, then maternal filicide rates would be far higher and the amount of overall deaths would likewise be higher. PND may be a contributing factor in the reason for some murderers, but it is not the cause in and of itself. There are a whole host of other factors that lead to catastrophic results such as murder. Looking at these factors as a whole is important; picking out just one is misleading. And not only is it misleading but it is unhelpful. It would be like treating a broken leg exclusively with pain relief. It would not work because pain is not the only issue. The bone needs to be set and stabilised, or further complications will result.

Constantly using PND as the reason for murders further stigmatises an already vulnerable group of women and makes people less likely to come forward, as they know that they will be judged as violent psychopaths who cannot be trusted with their own children. This fear of losing their kids stops many women from seeking help early on. Let's stop the false stereotype.

Furthermore, most people, when able to give a reason for the murder, cited loss of control as the reason which implies a psychotic break. A psychotic break that could well happen on top of PND, but PND is not necessarily dissociative and lacking in control. So again, other factors need to be examined. What pushed them over the edge isn't as simple as a single diagnosis of PND but involves all the other factors around it. In the vast majority of cases, it is how these factors interact rather than a single element.

If you think I'm harping on about nothing when it comes to the negative connotations placed upon PND sufferers, I'll quickly share a personal anecdote with you. Just prior to the Nikat case, another Australian toddler died at the hands of his mother. His name was Braxton, and his mother was Jasmine Mossman-Riley. Mossman-Riley, having left a suicide note on Facebook, jumped off a cliff in Maroubra whilst holding her son. It was tragic. Any death is tragic, more so a child's, and even more so when that child has the terror and pain of witnessing someone that they love killing them. Mossman-Riley's family have said that she suffered from PTSD as a result of domestic violence and have urged victims to speak out and get help before it is too late. Nobody wants something like this to happen again.

A family member of mine, on hearing about this case, decided to take me aside at the next family function and tell me that she had read about the mother in Sydney who had jumped off a cliff with her child and that the mother who jumped had PND, and I also had PND, and that I was to call her before I did something like that... blinks.... It was mortifying. Let's not even get into the logistics of the situation. The idea that I could get myself, a four year old, and two-year-old twins off a cliff at the same time when I struggle to merely get them in the car at the same time without losing a sock somewhere boggles the mind. A friend told me to shake it off, that she's just an older lady concerned about the kids. But why? Because there's a subconscious bias that PND equals potential baby killer, and not in the same way that anybody could become a killer. People link the two closely. It's a subconscious bias that needs to be challenged because it is not at all helpful.

Those who follow my blog know that I'm open about my struggles with PND. Heck, I've popped out this eBook all about it, and I blogged whilst in a psychiatric hospital, yet I have never written about an urge to hurt any of my children or kill them. That's because I've never had one. Sure, there have been times during the crying from painful reflux when I wished the crying would stop, but I blamed myself for not being a good enough mother, not the baby. I'm a living, breathing human being, not some blown-up stereotype created by the media, but an actual human being. Which means I don't fit into this bizarre mythos that has been made up about a fairly common condition. Evidently, that family member hasn't taken a gander at my blog. It was hurtful to be treated as a stereotype rather than a person. To be thought of as a caricature and not as who I really am. As if any time somebody murdered their child, I would be thought of and that other mums, just struggling to get by, and doing their absolute best, would be thought of as well. When I spoke to my friends who had also suffered from PND, they all shared similar stories of being shamed. After how hard we tried to be the best mums possible, in the end we were all just cut down to mindless killing machines because nothing else matters but that one label–PND. A label that shouldn't even mean "psychotic baby killer" in the first place. It was insensitive, and it hurt. And the irony is that, in this case, the media had reported that the mother suffered from post-traumatic stress disorder from domestic violence, not postnatal depression. And who really knows what the truth of the matter was? All we know is that a beautiful mother and her baby are gone and that they are missed, and we all wish they were back on Earth with us.

Conservative estimates state that approximately 1 in 7 mothers experience postnatal depression. That's just over 14%. Other figures have the rates considerably higher, even up to 30%. That's a lot of women. If you know 7 mothers, chances are at least one of them has experienced postnatal depression. They probably haven't even told you about it because of the stigma surrounding it. You will have thought the vast majority of them were excellent mothers with good relationships with their children. You'd think that because the vast majority of them are. Depression is not the same as being a pathological killer. It is not the same as not knowing wrong from right. It is not the same as being utterly unable to control your actions. It can be debilitating; it can cause bonding issues, but not always.

It does cause high levels of anxiety around your ability to parent. Anxiety that can interrupt sleep even more so than a baby up all night with reflux, or even twins with reflux. I've had both, the singleton and the twins with reflux. And I've also had postnatal depression. And yet I have never had an urge to hurt, maim, or murder, any one of my children. Commit suicide? Oh yeah, I've contemplated that. But murdering another human being, one utterly dependent on me? No, I have not. And, chances are, the women that you know with PND, regardless of if they have told you they have it or not, also aren't ticking time bombs just waiting to go off and kill a child. What they need is support, not fear.

Beyond postnatal depression is postnatal psychosis. Most cases are diagnosed within two weeks of birth. In this state, mothers do lose contact with reality and experience impaired decision-making capabilities. Unsupported women with this condition can cause serious damage before they receive help. Supported women in treatment usually have successful recoveries with meaningful relationships with their children. When I was in the Mother and Baby unit at a psychiatric hospital, I met four women who had been diagnosed with this condition. All four were picked up almost immediately after birth. Two had actually been booked into the hospital immediately before the birth because they had a history of dissociative mental illness. The first women I met with postnatal psychosis had been in treatment for three months by the time I met her. I would not have realised that she had a serious condition because her treatment had been so successful. I had noted that she did try to avoid being alone with her baby and had thought it was because she was a young mum who was simply anxious. Her anxiety was a whole other level because she still didn't quite trust herself. She loved her baby very much and did not have murderous intent. Then why was she worried? Perhaps explaining what the fourth woman I met with postnatal psychosis was like might help because she had only just been admitted when I met her. She had lost touch with reality and at times didn't seem to realise that her baby was her own. Had she been left alone with her baby, she could have left it on the side of the street, thinking it was a garbage bag or tossed it into the washing machine, thinking the baby was laundry. A pretty terrifying prospect for a mother to think she might harm her baby without realising.

I hope all of these women are doing great now. I know they were in the best place to recover and to embark upon a fantastic future. I'd also like to note that none of these women killed their babies. A diagnosis of postnatal psychosis on its own does not a killer make. A whole series of negative circumstances surrounding a mental-health issue generally contributes to a disastrous result such as murder, not simply the diagnosis of PND or PNP. The lack of support for these conditions is just as crucial as the condition itself. Be careful when using a label of mental illness to explain murder because there is far more to it than that, and you're unintentionally vilifying a group of vulnerable people who are far more likely to be the victims of crime than have committed one.

You know what I'd really love? If we started being more careful about what we assume about others because of one of the many "labels" that they "wear." And don't treat a bunch of anxious mums trying to do their best as unhinged murderers incapable of making a good decision. Just be nice to them. And I'd also like for the media to start reporting on the other factors that contribute to these tragic murders rather than sweeping them under the rug of PND. People really need to stop giving a simplistic diagnosis for a complex problem and stop further stigmatising anxious mums trying to do their best and already plagued with self-doubt. Give them support rather than judgment and false negative connotations. I get so tired of people thinking mental illness automatically explains murder. And there are so many different forms of mental illness that the term almost becomes useless as a descriptor when justifying an action. You need to at least start moving into subsets. It certainly takes more than depression to make a murderer out of a person, but all the other contributing factors rarely get a mention. It's just one factor, yet people just stop at mental illness as if that's enough and explains it all.

Now, I don't mean any of the above to suggest that we should automatically withdraw all empathy and support from accused killers and automatically assume that they're just plain evil. *Don't have empathy for people* is not the message that I wish to convey here at all. Have empathy, just don't randomly label people in order to express it. In fact, I lost a friend because we disagreed over a high-profile case involving an abandoned baby. My friend said this woman was a dog that deserved to be put down. I felt a slightly more compassionate approach needed to be taken until all the details were in. Maybe she was pure evil, but maybe she wasn't.

In November of 2014, a newborn was left in drain for six days in Quakers Hill. The baby was only one day old. The baby's thirty-year-old mother dropped the baby approximately 2.5 metres down a drain, an almost certain death sentence. It was horrifying. I think everyone in Australia just wanted to hug that baby. This incredible baby managed to survive for six days after being thrown out as if it were garbage. That baby was the ultimate fighter. People desperately tried to find the hospital that the little boy was in so that they could donate clothes and money to assure him the bright future he deserved. There was a very public outcry about the situation. People were calling for the mother to be locked up, beaten, and dumped in a drain in searing temperatures. It was a horrific situation, and people had an extreme reaction. It didn't surprise me one bit. All these strangers reacting strongly just proved how much they loved children. The threats, although vile and misguided, proved how precious the general public felt a child's life is. That's actually a good thing. We're moving away from thinking children should be seen and not heard and that we are entitled to beat them for minor infractions. In a way, this is progress.

However, the bit that not only surprised me but also disappointed me was that a woman I knew, who, like me, suffered from postnatal depression was calling the mother of this child all sorts of names, baying for her blood and saying how they couldn't comprehend what she had done and that she deserved no understanding. Now I've personally never had any urges to harm my children, nor have I had any dissociative breaks, which would make me a violent threat to others. I know right from wrong. But I felt that if we couldn't have compassion, or at least a willingness to withhold judgement until all the facts were out, for mothers who have done something so clearly out of the ordinary, then... well... who the fuck could?

I never tried to commit suicide with postnatal depression. I thought about it at length, but in the end, I never did because it was something that would deeply scar and traumatise my kids for the rest of their lives. I would leave them with a lifetime of issues requiring therapy. I simply could not put my kids through that. My suicide would be an even bigger issue than my crazy-arsed self hanging around. However, I withheld judgement from a friend who had attempted such things, multiple times and even when her children were in the home. I know what it's like to feel as if you're such a toxic person that your children would be better off without you. So I generally offer mothers who attempt suicide compassion because I know, sometimes, it is so damned hard to stay alive.

Make no mistake, the consequences for their children would be horrible, yet I still offer compassion. Sure, I could tell them they're awful and that they don't deserve kids and get up on my high horse and really go to town on them about how much damage they would do, but I don't. Why? Because I know what pain and confusion feel like, even if I have never gone through with any attempts at suicide. The same goes for mothers who leave their kids. I'm very much with my three babies. Mumma isn't going anywhere, save ill health (I can't rule out being hospitalised with pancreatitis again; unfortunately, I just have a bad pancreas that confounds the medical world). But I understand the urge to run because you feel as if you're not doing anything right, and your kids would be better off without you. Of course that's not true; they'll likely feel abandoned and unloved, but perception and reality don't always match up. In rare cases some kids are mildly relieved, but generally that parent has been abusive, and that child will still wear the scars, regardless.

I felt that as sufferers of depression, we should at least consider the possibility that the mother of the baby in Quakers Hill may not have abandoned this child into a filthy hole in hellish temperatures, which would almost certainly result in death, because she was evil but because she thought it'd be better for the child to die than be with her. It was still a horrible prospect but at least worth considering. I felt that we should at least consider the thought that her self-loathing wasn't merely to a depressive level but had moved into a psychotic state. What if she did this out of sick, depraved love, not because she was "a dog" or a "selfish mole" or any other insult levelled at her?

My compassion didn't make my heart break any less for that baby. I still wanted to hug that baby and make everything better for him. It didn't make his circumstances any less horrific. He was dropped into filth, where he was unlikely to ever be found, with no milk or hugs. Nothing can make that okay. The torment that sweet baby endured for six days when it so desperately needed love and nurturing sickened me. Not just a bit but to the point where I literally threw up. But I was willing to see that the mother might have needed help. That her mind was probably just as disgusting as that drain and that it needed to be cleaned out. She may not have necessarily been some demon that needed to be hung. So I withheld judgement on the mother.

I also think what some people fail to realise is that some women in the depths of postnatal psychosis, which usually happens early after birth, and this baby was dropped a day after his birth, can become so detached from reality that they just don't even recognise their baby as a baby. It is very rare, but as I previously mentioned, I have witnessed a woman being shown her baby and repeatedly refusing the baby and asking the nurses what the hell they were talking about. Thankfully, the baby was in a hospital, and the nurses were there to protect it whilst this woman went through her break from reality, but she could have so easily dumped her baby on the side of the street, not even realising what she had done. Should medical staff have failed to pick up on the situation early enough, then I could have very easily been reading a horror story about her instead of seeing her return to herself. And that's pretty scary to think.

But as I keep on saying, most mental illnesses on their own are not enough to turn someone into a murderer. It's just one possible factor. Heck, mental illness seems to also be a linking factor of creative types, so maybe we should just automatically assume all people with PND are going to become musicians or comedians instead of child killers. That would be nice. "Oh, you have PND—you must be so creative, and I look forward to your, no doubt, forthcoming compilation." Why aren't people assuming that we're all going to be literary greats like Virginia Woolf and Sylvia Plath, or blockbuster authors like J. K. Rowling or Patricia Cornwell? People rarely jump to the good associations; they go straight to the negative and icky ones. Pffft, I say, pfffft! In fact, it reminds me of a confrontation that I should have had when I first exited the madhouse.

The Mad Robin in the Attic

Let's get back to something a bit lighter than dead babies. How about we explore that link between creativity and being bat shit instead? I like having a bit of a write, and evidently a lot of a rant. In my adult life, I've now written my self-published serial *What Happens in Book Club...*, two unpublished children's fantasy novels, and most recently, this awesome collection that you're reading right now. You're welcome, Earth. Add to that the three fabulous novels I wrote in primary school, viciously slammed by the critics—siblings can be so cruel—but take it from me, they were sensational, and I'm quite the novelist. So it surprised me somewhat when I told a friend that I had been working on a "true fiction" inspired by my time in the nuthouse and they responded by saying, "Oh, are you still writing? I thought you'd give up now that you'd spent time in a psychiatric hospital. Wouldn't you be unpublishable now?"

. . .

. . .

. . .

WHAT THE ACTUAL EFF?!

I responded with something resembling a sentence and then disengaged from the conversation as soon as was politely acceptable. Perhaps not even as soon as was politely possible. I went a bit "deer in the headlights" and just ran for the exit when I saw the opportunity. Clearly, they were unfamiliar with Susanna Kaysen and the now famous quote from *Girl, Interrupted*, "Don't point your finger at crazy people." Admittedly, I didn't explode or bark or start wailing or use too many *ors* in a sentence or forget to use commas.... I just muttered something about liking writing and then retreated to the blanket fort in my head. It was warm and cosy there, and I received plenty of imaginary pats on my head. But in hindsight, I should have schooled this person on the fact that being a bit on the cray cray side should not be viewed as a hindrance to creative endeavours. Here's what I should have said:

In 1979 two great things happened, I was born (shamelessly arrogant but I feel the sense of drama was required), and *The Madwoman in the Attic* was first published. *The Madwoman in the Attic* was possibly my favourite text that I studied in university. And you, *good sir,* should read it. Because not only would you lock away the "madwoman" in literature but also in society. As soon as a woman is counter to your understanding, she is to be boxed up and put away. Did it not occur to you that not all who seek help are snivelling, messy haired, violent psychopaths? That we can be productive members of society? That perhaps the locking away and stigmatising of the "madwoman" is what forces them into violent gibberhood.

And so what if I am a crackpot? At least I am in good company! Sylvia Plath, Anne Sexton, Virginia Woolf, Luanne Rice, Elizabeth Wurtzel, Suzanna Kaysen, and Patricia Cornwell have all been considered raving loonies at some point. They've all spent time in "supportive environments whilst they recovered from exhaustion." So when you think about it, being barking mad would pretty much be a prerequisite. If anything, I should be expecting a bunch of marauding female novelists to come barging through my door at any given moment in order to clutch me to their collective bosom and shower me with literary agents' contact details. I too am now a raving writer. I too drink tea as if it's on tap. Ich bin ein lunatic. And honestly what real writer doesn't have a scarf, a beret, and a jumbo-sized pack of antidepressants on them at all times? (I'm pretty sure I stole part of that quote from a joke about stereotypes made by *Destination Saigon* author, Walter Mason.) So just go take your snivelling comment and stuff it down your fluffy, lemon jumper.

Oh, on second thoughts, it's probably better that I didn't say that. Let's face it, if I did, he probably would have just said, "Yeah, that makes a lot of sense if you think about it like a crazy person."

As you might have noticed, I'm a bit obsessed with writers. Particularly Australian women writers. I obsess over them the same way most people do over actors and singers. I follow them on Facebook, I check their Twitter feeds daily, and I get excited if they happen to be running a workshop close to me that I can afford. And if you've followed my blog at all, you would know that one of my biggest lady writer crushes (LWC) is on Tara Moss. And I've actually found that my obsession helps me get through some of my tough days. Not because I'm procrastinating by cyber stalking them but because they inspire me.

My obsession with Tara Moss is so strong that I use expressions like, "I'm channelling my inner Moss," and, "I totally Mossed it," much to my friends' amusement. And I'll be honest—it has caught on with them too. Anytime we appear particularly serene and confident when under stress, we'll say, "I see you're Mossing it." If one of us is flipping out, we'll say, "What would Tara do? Put on her lipstick and pull herself together, damn it." I've actually started wearing red lipstick now. I had to go *emergency-purchase* it one stressful morning in order to "get on Moss of it," and I have never looked back. I own several red lipsticks now. Even though I have thin little lizard lips, I still rock that red. This switch to red lippy did come as a shock to people who have known me for years and are more familiar with me channelling my inner Virginia Woolf rather than Moss.

But you know what? It works. I feel much more confident with my lip mask on. So I drink a cup of tea, put on my lipstick and high heels, and I'm ready to face the day. Well, not every day. Let's be real; I'm probably sitting about in pyjama bottoms paired with a sweaty T-shirt and decaying grey slippers as you read this. But I do find "Mossing it" occasionally useful. However, I'll let you in on a little secret. Lean in closer, closer. I have to italicise it because this is such a secrety secret—*Tara Moss isn't the only person I channel.* Gasp. Yup. I'm a bit of a lady writer crush hussy (LWCH???). Although Tara Moss is my go-to at the moment, I can't solve all the world's problems through giving it "a red hot Moss." Here are some more LWC that I shall share with you so that you too can channel them in your hour of need.

What would Emily Maguire do? She'd put on her pyjamas and pull herself apart. Because sometimes you just need to get comfy in your sauce-stained pj's to truly become one with yourself. If she was scared of something, she'd go out and confront it. She'd research it, interview it, visit it—she'd get that business all taken care of because knowledge and understanding is power. Then she'd go home and get comfy. Because pyjamas are awesome.

What would Kate Forsyth do? Plaster on a smile, sip some champagne, and hug her many, many books, published in many, many countries. When you're as internationally recognised as Kate Forsyth, not much fazes you, so just drink champers and be fab. We all need to just shake it off with a champagne and a smile every now and then. If I was to channel pre-published Kate Forsyth (translation: broke), then to "Forsyth it" would mean to be focused, devoted, and without distractions or detractions. Choose your priorities and go with that. If that means skipping a few meals to do a writing course, then so be it. So really, however you "Forsyth it," pre-published or internationally celebrated, you'll be doing something pretty amazing. Self-belief is key.

What would Nakkiah Lui do? No idea; she's a bit like the Spanish Inquisition: nobody expects them. The only thing I know is that she'll challenge, she'll be unique, she'll probably swear, and she'll definitely make you laugh. If you want to "Lui it," you'll need to be able to think on your feet and always do the unexpected and *be* the unexpected. On a side note: I am glad she's on the TV show *Black Comedy* so that I can see her stuff more often. Selfish, I know, but I rarely get out to the theatre these days with three kids under primary-school age.

What would Margo Lanagan do? Something so profoundly brilliant that it beggars belief, and then she would be self-deprecating about it. Modesty, thy name is Margo Lanagan. Okay, I haven't channelled my inner Lanagan yet, because I haven't written anything as brilliant as her yet, but I look forward to the day I do, because then I'll be smug as hell instead of self-deprecating. I'm going to do it. Maybe.

What would Hannah Kent do? Start a bidding war over her first novel . . . shit! I forgot to do that. Wow, this is starting to get depressing. Let's move on, people.

What would Anita Heiss do? Be groundbreaking, brilliant, devoted, and still be family oriented. She gets her PhD and still writes in a genre some people think is beneath them, chick lit, because she is incredible and doesn't let anyone dictate to her what is important. I feel brave and powerful just saying her name out loud. I hope my daughter channels her inner Heiss when she grows up. Mummy will always be here; please don't forget me.

What would Pamela Freeman do? Say something sassy as hell and make everyone laugh, then follow it up with a ridiculously insightful comment. Pamela is cheeky, she's funny, she's willing to tease her writer friends on panels just to make them laugh, and she follows it up with intellectual insights. She writes across different genres and different age groups despite so many people in the publishing industry trying to dictate that you can only do one thing. She is 100% her own woman. In short, she's as close as you can get to a Terry Pratchett witch in real life. Just say what you want, write what you want, and be who you want, because that's what Pamela would do.

What would Kerri Sackville do? She'd eat some Nutella and write a poem about wine . . . because sometimes we all need to do that.

So when I'm feeling down, I just channel one of my heroes. I put on the performance of the quality that they represent to me and I fake it until I make it. These people work for me because I am obsessed with writers. I should really talk to my therapist about this. But they might not work for you because your hobbies are probably different than mine. I'd recommend picking strong women in a field that you're interested in and using them as your go-to for inspiration on hard days. Sure, it would be nice to think we're all so well adjusted that we can conquer every mountain without any help, but some days, we're just not feeling it. Get a little motivation bank of people and characteristics you admire. Perform them until they become natural to you. Being a magnificent, well-adjusted babe doesn't come naturally to all of us. Some of us really do have to fake it until we make it. And that's okay.

Excuse me, but I need to go have a break and contemplate why on Earth I think I am at all qualified to be giving tips to anyone else. What would Robin do? Freak the fuck out and then post some Tweet about her bowel movements. Should she really be giving advice to anyone?

Play to Your Strengths

During my time on the inside, I had learned that when you're in the grips of a mental illness such as depression or anxiety, you can begin to lose yourself, especially when you're a mother. You put so much energy into just getting the day-to-day tasks, of keeping your kids alive and building their self-esteem, that you just want to crash and burn at the end of the day. The idea of doing something as trivial as treating yourself seems like way too much effort when you're so desperate to sleep. And to be honest, "treating" yourself with trivial things probably isn't worth it. But you do need to do something for yourself. You can't just keep on giving out joy to your children if you don't have something inspiring you on the inside. Yes, your children's love is precious and does stoke the furnace, but you also need something for you. Everybody needs a space where they can decompress and just be themselves and not a servant to anyone else. No matter how cute the master is. For some people, they lose themselves in art. They set aside half an hour either early in the morning, or in the evening, and they just create with abandon. For others, it can be knitting awesome creations; for some, it's building up a financial empire; for me, it is writing. I have always loved writing and finding a space for doing it is imperative to my happiness. The group therapist who told me to just stop writing until my kids got older was so wrong. How much writing I'm doing is like a litmus test for my mental health. She may as well have told a guitar player to cut off one of their hands until their kids got older.

 I think my love of literature was inspired by the word "bum." As a child, I adored the word. I would use it ad nauseam. I could turn every conversation back to "bum," in particular, bear or bare bum. For example, "What are you watching?" – "Play School. Little Ted has a bear bare bum." Champagne comedy. My mother, on the other hand, was not overly fond of the word. I must confess that she still is not. She felt it was most unbecoming of a young lady and tried to think of various other things I could say instead. All to no avail; "bum" was the word I loved. And still love. The most success my mother had was after one of my siblings had dropped the c-bomb (yes, *the* c-bomb), and my mother trotted out that tired old adage, "If you don't know what it means, don't say it." I chimed in with how I knew what a bum was and proceeded to define it at length. So my mother told me, "If you don't know how to spell it, then don't say it."

This statement had no logic, if this was the case then all I could really say at the time was my name, and if I refused to say anything except for my name then I would get into trouble for being rude. However, it still stumped me. I studied the alphabet on my wall for quite some time and then finally burst out of my room yelling, "BUM! I can say it! B.U.M." My mother, rather than falling over herself congratulating me for my exceptional development in literacy, was not impressed at all. In fact, she simply sniffed and walked away, shooting a withering glare over her shoulder. For the next few months, I proceeded to tell every single person that I encountered that I knew how to spell bum and then spelled it for them. Be careful what you say to your children; it does not always quite work out as you'd wish. My mother did not clasp her hands in delight and squee over how clever I was at this point either. Unbelievable! However, I think if it was not for this overwhelming need to uncover the mystery of the word "bum," then I possibly would not have then started searching for new words. Truly, "bum" inspired my love of words. I am well aware that this is not the typical genesis story that writers share, but I feel as if we're friends now and that I can be honest. Brava for bum.

By the time I was ten, I had progressed past the word "bum." I was able to spell other words too. Not brilliantly. I'm dyslexic, so there's never any guarantee that what I'm thinking is what will end up on the page. It's kind of like a lucky dip. An embarrassing lucky dip where grammar Nazis mock you for being you. Which kind of sucks and hurts my feelings. But as per usual, I have digressed. Perhaps I should have called this *Digressions of a Mad Mooer*. Did we just come up with a name for a sequel? I think we did. Good job, us. Getting back to my literary chops, my first novel was a gripping fantasy adventure that covered multiple lands ranging from underwater worlds to forests to remote islands to places that existed in air breaches between land and water. It had it all. And I listed them all. Anyone who has done a writing course will know that this is a big no-no. You're supposed to show, not tell. But I was only ten.

But I was a ten year old who had read *Magician* by Raymond E Feist and *Spellsinger* by Alan Dean Foster. So in short, I was quietly confident that I knew what I was doing. It followed the journey of a sexy hobbit. Yes, I had also read the great Tolkien. I was and am a fantasy nerd, so of course I'd read Tolkien. I was pretty proud of the sexy hobbit, as that was one of my many points of difference that I thought would get the punters in. I'd learned from *Spellsinger* that people liked some hard loving in their stories, not just walking about with a bunch of dwarves. I called him Arti, and his mission was to stop the encroaching darkness with his trusty band of representatives from other species. Now, of course, there were lots of problems with the girls fighting over Arti because he was just so gosh-darned sexy. He was so sexy that he almost disrupted the wedding of the fairy king's daughter because how could she possibly resist him? And, of course, his generally being so darned appealing caused all sorts of problems with pretty much every other male character because they were so jealous of him. I know what you're thinking: please publish this magnificent epic now. Love stories, darkness, a varied setting—what more could you want?

Thoughtful names? Well I had those too. I made extensive use of my thesaurus. Clearly, I was ahead of my time, as that has become all the rage since *Fifty Shades of Grey*. At ten, I could have been the next E. L. James. I have wasted my fucking life. One of the characters, who was a cross between Tolkien's Gandalf and Feist's Macros the Black, was named Callow Erudite. Now these seemed like totally fine words for names to me at the time because I hadn't really heard them before, and so assumed nobody else would have either. He was an old and wise magician who looked extremely young. He was guarded by a shape-shifting gargoyle. Or was it a griffin? Something "g" related. As you can clearly see, I had it all. Just one problem: my public, AKA my family, simply could not get to the blistering sexual magnetism of Arti, nor the rich tapestry that was the land, and they certainly didn't encounter the carefully planned characters because they refused to read past the introduction.

After my brother picked himself up off the ground from laughing hysterically, I wouldn't be surprised to learn that a small amount of wee snuck out. My brother tried to be tactful and offer suggestions. Stupid things like, although I had lots of things in my novel, did I have to list every single one of them in my prologue? Couldn't I just wait for them to be introduced in the story? *But then how would the reader know just how great this book would be unless I put it in the world's longest and most detailed list ever right at the start of the novel?* Duh! I refused to take on any suggestions. I knew better. I was ten and utterly brilliant. I'd written a novel—what was his greatest achievement at the time? Finishing his school certificate? Constantly topping English? Becoming dux repeatedly? In hind sight he might have been onto something. Here's my prologue.

Prologue

This story was set long ago, long before there were humans. It was a set in time when, Banshees, Behemoths, Centaurs, Cerberuses, Cyclopses, Dark Elves, Demons, Dragons, Druids, Dwarves, Enchanters, Fairies, Fays, Feys, Forest Elves, Furies, Gargoyles, Ghouls, Giants, Gnomes, Goblins, Gremlins, Griffins, Gypsies, Hags, Halflings, Hermits, Hobbits,

Hobgoblins, Imps, Lemures, Mages, Magicians, Medusas, Mermaids, Minotaurs, Monsters, Muses, Necromancers, Ogres, Orcs, Pegasuses, Phantoms, Phoenixes, Pirates, Pixies, Poltergeists, Prophets, Sirens, Sorceresses, Spectres, Sprites (water, earth, fire, and air sprites), Star Elves, Trolls, Unicorns, Vipers, Warlocks, Werewolves, Witches, Wraiths, and talking animals roamed the earth.

Just quietly; for the love of all things sacred, nobody ever tell Raymond E Feist or Alan Dean Foster about my brilliant tribute. I am still obsessed with them both and should I ever be in the same area as them, I would like to get a book signed by them. I'll have to buy new ones because the many, many copies I have are in a somewhat fragile state after being loved pretty much to death. When I ask them to sign my chest—I mean "novel"—I'd like them not to say, "That name… why is it so familiar? Oh, you're her. You're Sexy Hobbit Lady." Give a fellow nerd a break, and let's just keep this between ourselves.

Even as an adult, I still love fantasy stories. I think I use it as a form of escapism, regardless of if I am reading them or writing them. They help keep me somewhat sane when I just need to give myself a break from the real world, and they also give me hope. They give me heroes that overcome insurmountable odds. They show me that the human spirit can overcome. Even when my daughter was in her spica cast and I was barely sleeping, I still wrote fantasy. I needed the escape. I needed to be in a world where better treatments than spica casts were used for hip dysplasia. So I came up with a novel set 1000 years in the future about a little girl whose hips were out of phase. Her condition was known as hip dysphasia. She wasn't hampered by a plaster cast but had a light weight exoskeleton around her legs until her hips phased properly. Going into that world helped me cope with a situation that was almost utterly unbearable for me. I didn't have to write a journal to help me cope; I had to write an escape. A nice place to hang out where awful stuff wasn't happening. So I wrote a lighthearted children's novel. Here's how the first chapter of *Chloe Prime: Alien Space Vet* goes.

> BANG!
> Chloe Prime poked her head out above her blankets and eyed her wardrobe suspiciously. Had it just made a noise? She watched and waited for a few minutes. Nothing. Perhaps it had all been in her

imagination. A flight of fancy? She nestled back under her covers.

BANG!

Chloe pulled her covers down again and glared at her wardrobe. Honestly, this was getting ridiculous. She had to get a good night's sleep for the first day at her new school tomorrow. This just would not do.

BANG!

Chloe vaulted out of bed and stood in front of her wardrobe in a fighting stance. Her hair reared out from her head in crazy curls, ready for action. Her legs were encased in a metallic exoskeleton, which made her look every bit like a miniature cyborg, with medusa hair, at the ready. If there was a monster in that wardrobe, she was going to have at it.

"I came here for a bedtime story and to kick butt," ten-year-old Chloe challenged her empty cupboard. "And I already finished my story."

Whoosh!

Kent Prime came running into his daughter's room, closely followed by her mother. Chloe turned to see her father staring at her in shock.

"Monsters, Dad," Chloe quickly informed her father. "In the cupboard. I've got them pinned."

Kent Prime attempted to move further into the room.

"Get back!" Chloe yelled. "It's too dangerous! Save Mum."

Chloe's father laughed and closed the gap between them, scooping up his daughter.

"There are no monsters here, Little Miss Lady."

"Are you nervous about school tomorrow?" Chloe's mother asked.

"What?" Chloe snorted in surprise. "I'm excited about school. I just happen to have a rather serious monster problem to deal with."

"I'll deal with any monsters," Chloe's father said. "You just go to bed. Besides, you know that they're more scared of you than you are of them."

"But Dad, what if there are ghosts, or fairies... or I heard that sometimes little time-travelling pirates come breaking down your..." Chloe began.

"No buts, no brownies, no bandits! You need your rest if you're going to be on the school shuttle on time tomorrow morning," Kent Prime tutted. "Besides, you know all our wardrobes are double coated with Kevlarized Graphene. Nothing is getting through."

"But what about bears? You know . . . sort of hiding in the cupboard rather than coming through it?" Chloe was grasping at straws. She knew she would never win this argument, and she was getting quite tired anyway. Her mother kissed her good-night.

"Don't you worry about any bears, sweetie," Mum said as she walked out of the room. "I'm sure you can just talk your way out of trouble without fighting."

Chloe shrugged doubtfully but cuddled up to her teddy Sinbad and began dozing off with images of swashbuckling bears, whispering to fairy ghosts, in her head.

TAP TAP TAP

At this point, Chloe leapt out of her bed and flung her cupboard open.

SQUEAK!

"You! What are you doing in there? You know you're not supposed to come inside."

Squeak, squeak, squeak?

"Oh all right. I'll see if I can sneak into the kitchen and find you something, but then you really must go outside."

Squeak.

"Yes, I know mice don't really love cheese."

Squeak, squeak?

"No you can't come. Mum will freak if she sees a mouse in the kitchen."

I know that it doesn't begin with a brilliant prologue that lists all the species to come, but I became so enchanted with this little world that this safe haven from hip dysplasia soon blew out into a plan for seven novels. I've even drafted the first two. It's just nice to be in a world free of that kind of suffering. There are few things worse than seeing your child in pain. Sure, this world has its own complications, and the characters face hardships, but hip dysplasia and putting people into traction isn't one of them. Writing helped me keep on going when I felt as if I had reached my end point.

Now for you it doesn't have to be writing. You may not have been quite as taken with the word "bum" as I was. I can't imagine why not, but there's no accounting for taste in some people. Even if you don't write, you do have to do something for you that suits you. Play to your strengths. If you're great at sports, then join a team. If you love writing, do a writing course. If you love doodling, get some adult colouring books. Just do something for you. Something meaningful. Something more meaningful than just eating a chocolate. Because eating a chocolate is fun, but you can do that hiding in a cupboard whilst the kids are awake. Give yourself "you" time. Real "you" time, where you feed your soul.

Impractical Parenting

A while back in Australia, there was an advert for a "stress protect" deodorant. I would watch those ads with much envy. The woman portrayed in this ad was so incredibly gorgeous with one of those smiles that made you feel as if she was emitting sunshine from her very being. The ad depicted a beautiful, happy, well dressed, and organised mother who was able to juggle her job and her toddler with ease. She looked exactly like the type of mum who has time to brush her hair every single day. The kind of mum who goes to the toilet on her own. In short, a total mole that I was deeply jealous of. Oh, how I longed to be her. Now I know better.

During that same time frame that this ad was airing, I used to walk around Darling Harbour, with my twins in their pram and my then three year old on my back in an ergo, daily. I'd think of that woman and how much I wanted to be her, looking fresh and fancy-free. Flicking my hair and laughing. But one day as sweat dripped down my butt crack as I was pushing the twins and lugging about my toddler, I thought, "Screw you, stress protect woman. You've got nothing on me."

And honestly, she's got nothing on any real mum. Sure, in the ad she's walking about looking all fresh faced and beautiful, but she's doing it with one happy kid, a phone, and a bag of groceries; that's it. Let's see her do it with one *hangry* kid, her work on the phone telling her that her miscarriage is inconvenient to them because now she won't be on maternity leave (not that I'm bitter and still mad three years later, mofos), plus groceries in a broken bag, the toddler's discarded shoes tucked under her armpit along with a million other things the toddler has produced from seemingly nowhere, and a husband who turns up after the witching hour is over and is all like, "What's your problem? Kids are fun; it's not work." Now, that's when you need stress protection. I want to see a mum with messy hair, being yelled at by an army of hangry kids, on the verge of developing an eye twitch, and then someone walks up and says, "My goodness, you look atrocious, but boy, do you smell fresh. What deodorant are you using?" Not a mum on an easy day, a day when she's returning home with her happy kid with the groceries whilst having a chat on the phone with a girlfriend to find her husband home from work early. Because that's a good day, not a stress-protection worthy day. Oh my goodness, that got angry so quickly.

I think what writing my confessions has shown me is that I am so wise. Oh so very wise. And I should, in fact, write my own parenting book. Sure, I have no qualifications as a paediatrician, paediatric nurse, early childhood teacher etc., but why should that make me any less of an expert? So let me share some of my best parenting tips with you. I shall start with how to handle a triple nappy change. I had three kids in nappies all at the same time, so this is a situation that I know all too well. Just make sure you follow these four steps in order; otherwise, they won't work effectively, and you might have an embarrassing mishap. I'd hate for that to happen to anyone but myself.

> Step 1: Get twin A, open nappy, stick baby's foot in poo; when jingling the baby awkwardly in an attempt to clean foot, smear poo all over changing table, mop up poo, get urinated on whilst distracted by poo, place baby on a play mat to avoid baby getting further soaked again, have baby pee again, quickly put on nappy, and move onto another play mat with twin B—you have a million play mats because everyone gave you one. Finish dressing baby A.

Step 2: Change twin B next to twin A on play mat, as all other surfaces are urine and poop soaked. Open nappy; twin A sticks hand in twin B's nappy— clean off twin A's hand. Whilst cleaning twin A, twin B is to power spew all over himself and twin A. Changing the clothes of both twins, two year old to rip off nappy—remind two year old to use potty if they need to wee. The two year old is to tell you it's okay, that they can just wee on the ground and crouches to urinate on ground.

Step 3: Put nappy on two year old, two year old immediately does massive poo, chase two year old around the house whilst they scream, "no poo, no nappy change," eventually subdue two-year-old terrorist, and change nappy whilst you contemplate how the poo has managed to defy time, space, gravity, and sanity.

Step 4: Drink a soothing cup of tea whilst developing an eye twitch and thinking about newspapering your whole house.

Don't worry. I have so much more to give, like how to deal with three kids crying at once... it's called vodka. Vodka is actually one of the unsung heroes of motherhood. I actually referred to it in an article I wrote about cleaning. If my mother-in-law is reading this, her head possibly exploded at the thought of me writing an article about cleaning tips, but it's true. I did. I once applied for a job as a writer for one of those mummy websites. They set a topic for the application, and I wrote to it. They actually told me that they loved my article, that they were in the process of putting on a new editor, and hiring me would be at the top of their list of things to do once that position had been filled. I never heard back from them again. Even when I subsequently asked about how the search for the new editor was going and tried to make some polite inquiries. They blanked me. Perhaps they discovered some photos of my home and could see that I was not indeed practicing what I preached. So here was the article that got such a positive response within minutes of it being emailed off, then blanked forevermore afterwards.

How to Clean up Wall Art

"If you have got a budding Picasso on your hands, then chances are you have experienced artistic expressions that you and your wall did not appreciate. No need to tear your own ear off with madness, wondering what to do, because these tried-and-true methods will get you through your artistic crises.

Baby Wipes

This is an absolute go-to for all concerns in life; from pooey bottoms to stained wedding dresses, the humble baby wipe is the first point of call. And now it can be used on your walls too. I prefer *Huggies* because they're thicker and more durable, but some of my friends swear by *Johnson & Johnson* unscented, and others feel *Wotnot* wipes makes them feel as if they are being less of an environmental terrorist. Whatever your preference, they're all good, really.

Bi-Carb and White Vinegar

If the humble nappy wipe has let you down, there is always the bicarb/white vinegar mix, great for cleaning ovens, dishwashers, and apparently walls. Mix vinegar and bicarb into a paste, then scrub at the art in circular motions with a toothbrush. If you're feeling a little saucy add the juice of half a lemon to give your walls that fun and fresh fragrance. I'll be honest: I am yet to find this method to work on stubborn wall "art," but my friends all swear by it.

Chux Magic Eraser

Where have you been all my life? The supermarket, apparently, for under $5. This gets off crayon. As any proud mother to an emerging artist knows, crayon is the worst for getting off walls. I had scrubbed my walls with all manner of gel bleaches, toothpastes, and tough stain removal sprays until I discovered the *Chux Magic Eraser*. It is a godsend. It can leave faint residue of the crayon colour on the wall, but, of course, you've got baby wipes handy to finish the job.

WD-40

There are some stains on this Earth that even the *Chux Magic Eraser* cannot defeat. Certain types of crayons and paints have major sticking power; that's when you need to bring out the big guns. *WD-40*. Just make sure you open all the windows to avoid fumigating yourself… although after dealing with all that art, you may want to get a little fumed. You can pick it up from any hardware store for under $10.

The Drastic Three

If none of the above has worked, then you are left with only three choices.

1. Vodka–apply directly to lips
2. Frame it; pretend you're living in the Sistine Chapel
3. Move house

Nine out of ten of my friends prefer option 1. Nine out of ten of my friends may have a drinking problem.

I stand by the "Drastic Three." I am seriously contemplating "3" myself. Tell your friends to buy my shit; I need moving money! Okay, so it might be a little over the top, and there might be a couple of people out there who might not want to use my "methods" of nappy changing or cleaning. Perhaps I'm not some glamorous home expert in the making ready to have people hanging on my every word.

I think the twins were about nine months old when it became abundantly clear that my life would never be glamorous enough for a Hollywood-style reality television program nor would I be taken seriously enough to be a parenting expert. Not that I'd ever dreamed of such things, really. I can barely tell myself what to do, let alone others. Here's a snapshot of one morning after my oldest had just turned three. (Let's see if you can pick exactly why my parenting tips will never take off as endorsed by anybody, including myself, nor will a made-for-television biopic be made about me.)

One of the twins woke up crying at around 6 am. It was the youngest, by a minute. I'm not going to insult your intelligence and pretend I don't know which one it was and that they both do it all the time. The baby of the family does not love sleep. Neither does the oldest child; it was driving me crazy. I should say crazier. My husband looked at me sleepily, saying how exhausted he was, and so I lovingly attempted to kick him the heck out of bed because I had already been up all night with one of the twins (yes, the baby of the family), and I was exhausted. There was no sexy lingerie, and not even the exciting conflict of a swearing match because I was too zombified to do much but grunt angrily and flail a foot at the husband's tail.

The husband got up, did not pick up the crying twin (yes, yes, it was the baby of the family), and get this: he sits on the toilet. He stays there for like an hour. Who does that? So I managed to pry my eyes open and stumble out of bed, because you can't just leave babies crying. Particularly not ones with reflux, because they vomit everywhere. I collected the babies in my arms, then heard the toddler monkey calling out in her dulcet tones for love. Translation: she was screaming like a banshee. I ducked into her room, she jumped on my back, and I carried all three children into the lounge room. Just a reminder, the husband is still on the toilet.

I changed the twins' nappies and managed not to get poo everywhere. Mainly because they only did wees. The toddler asked where Daddy was. I told her that he was on the toilet. She nodded sagely and told me how much Daddy loved the toilet. I agreed. He still does. Always has, always will. At this point, I probably started daydreaming about going to the toilet on my own during the day. I enjoy these little delusions. They're like a little slice of heaven. This divine toilet daydream could be done as some sort of dreamscape in a telemovie. Perhaps they could do one of those foggy transitions and then some beautiful rose-coloured lighting as they focus on me sitting on the can. Every parent would get the pleasure of that.

After my toilet fantasies, I got the boys their bottles ready (at nine months, they were bottle fed; I guess that could have caused some controversy worthy of television. People could have come and had a breast-in at my front door, and I could have doused them with goat's milk or formula) whilst also getting my daughter a cup of milk at her desired temperature. The exact temperature still changes daily. She then asked for cake for breakfast. I said no. I think we all know that at that point, some ominous music would be needed. Nobody says no to a threenager and walks away unscathed.

Fortunately, the husband finally got off the loo, distracting the three year old from an almost certain meltdown. He told everyone about the quality of his poo and the effectiveness of his scissor bone. Nobody is going to be putting around memes of us saying "couple goals." Whatever. I gave the boys their bottles, and the satisfied husband made our daughter some toast. There was some father and daughter toast eating whilst she described how the world worked. Little insights such as if you get blue and gold paint and mix them, then you get green paint, but if you mix blue and gold glitter, you just get blue and gold glitter mixed together. True. Even at three, she knew what was what.

At this point, one of the twins vomited all over himself, his brother, and me. His brother laughed. Baby of the family, you are lucky your brother has a weird sense of humour. I put dripping wet boys onto a play mat, stripped them of their vomit-drenched wondersuits, and then slowly made my dripping way to the laundry to strip myself and dump my clothes in the laundry. My daughter, at some point, had escaped from breakfast land and found me and yelled, "Mummy is nudie." The husband wandered over and raised his eyebrows at me in a suggestive manner. A few weeks later when I complained that he never tells me I'm pretty, he said, "What about that time in the laundry?" Three young kids, and yet the romance is clearly still going strong in our household. #CoupleGoals

The husband then jumped in the shower. I swallowed my bitterness and went off into a fantasy land where I get to have showers too. This should bring on another transition and some funky lighting. Unfortunately, they'll have to use a shower model because me being in the shower is so rare that there is no file footage to use. I smell like a mouldy arse. No past tense necessary on that last sentence. I'm pretty sure this is just my life now.

I was drawn out of my hot and steamy fantasy land by what sounded like a flock of squawking seagulls coming from the lounge room. I entered the lounge room still naked—you're welcome, nosey neighbours—to discover that my daughter had left her toast on the ground, and the boys had fallen upon the unattended prey. One twin had a mammoth piece in his mouth, and the other was beating a smaller slice against the ground to ensure it was well and truly dead before he ate it. What can I say? I have little cave babies. It's like living with thunder personified.

It wasn't even 8 am at this point, but all the sex appeal had already been ripped from my day, so much so that I am even now in some kind of sexiness deficit. I'm pretty sure that most people want to get parenting advice from people who can manage to pee and shower. Perhaps my husband could become some sort of guru. After all, he does it all. He works, showers, pees, and has as many kids as I do. And as for Hollywood, well, their mums look like Mila Kunis, not flat chested, frizzy-haired thirty-seven year olds who need a good hot shower. This reminds me that I should probably wash my face and put on some moisturiser. It has been a couple of days. Beauty blogger is possibly also off my career list.

Maybe I could become a pregnancy expert to earn my new home? I've had three kids. One was via the vajayjay, and the other two babies came out through the sunroof. Surely that counts for something? And everybody wants to know how to have a fairy-tale pregnancy, and I definitely know a lot about fairy tales. I love fairy tales. One might even say I'm obsessed with them. So surely my combination of having had a kid or three and liking to read should impart me with some sort of expertise. I'm feeling good about this. I think we're onto something.

How to Have a Fairy Tale Pregnancy

<u>Wicked Step-Sisters</u>: Your family and the in-laws will go mental when you are pregnant, even more mental if they already

are mental. You'll have plenty of wicked comments and demands made.

Rapunzel: Let down your hair; sure, you'll have glossy hair on your head. It's one of the perks of pregnancy hormones. Unfortunately, you'll be a wildersavage all over. Who wants to bend and stretch over that bump to groom their nethers?

Sleeping Beauty: You'll be tired all through your first and third trimester and on top of that, you'll be gassy. So not only will you be sleepy, but everyone around you will be gassed into submission.

Wicked Step-Sisters: Fetch me my wig; people will suddenly need you to do everything for them, and the thought of losing you once the baby comes will bring out the clingy *me me me* attitude in everyone. You thought it would be joyous and bonding, but sadly some people are just selfish arseholes.

The Emperor's New Clothes: Don't worry about those new clothes. Go nude; it's too hot for anything else.

The Little Mermaid: You'll feel fat and cumbersome, even in aqua aerobics. It is actually way more like *The Little Whale*.

The Frog Prince: Your husband is a toad one minute, then a prince the next.

Cinderella: Scrub the floor; you'll want to clean everything, and anyone who gets in your way is the enemy. Stab them with a mop handle.

Jack and the Bean Stalk: Fi fi fo fum, I smell the blood of an English muffin. You will crave things, not necessarily weird things, probably just watermelon, but if you don't get it, you will hulk up.

Puss in Boots: Occasionally you'll insist on wearing high-heeled boots so you can be even hotter than those celebrity mums. It's your crazy pregnancy hormones talking; don't listen to them.

Snow White: Retreating to the woods for some time out probably isn't such a bad idea. But of course all those needy dwarves will track you down.

The Nightingale: If you are put on bed rest, you will go stir-crazy. That is all.

Fairest of Them All: Sure, your skin looks great; you've been sweating up a storm by vomiting all the time. Toxins don't have a chance to set in with you constantly doing the old heave ho.

On second thoughts, I'm possibly not entirely uplifting enough to be a pregnancy guru. I can be a bit of a stroppy cow, not just mad one. I can't even do those, "You know you're a mother when… you feel like you have multiple hearts, one for yourself and then one for each of your children," things properly. I'm more like:

You know you're a mother when…

- You run out of pads, so you use a nappy in the interim.
- You discover you haven't actually run out of pads, your brain was just too fried to see them, so now you're a grown woman wearing an infant boy's nappy for no reason.
- The idea of having a cocktail with the girls makes you so excited that you can't sleep… for the entire month beforehand, because that's how far in advance you have to arrange things.
- You've forgotten how to go to the toilet unsupervised.
- A good day is when you get to brush your teeth.
- One spew on your top isn't enough to make you change it.

- You enjoy snuggling in bed on your own even more than a university student.
- Your food intake is even worse than a university student's. It consists of half-sucked-on leftovers you have found on the floor.
- The idea of giving yourself a timeout is appealing.
- Having a headache is not an excuse; it's a way of life.
- The spirit is willing but the body is exhausted.
- Your partner's very presence infuriates you for no particular reason.
- You're always hungry but never get food because your children steal it.
- You think it's okay to sniff another human's butt.
- You think of creating a blanket fort and hiding in it on a regular basis.
- Chocolate is your bedfellow.
- Chocolate is also your closet fellow. And "wherever you can eat it hiding" fellow.
- Go to put laundry away, forget what you're doing, go to make a cup of tea, forget you made it, go to find clean clothes, can't find them, then drink cold tea you have just discovered.
- You ask your babysitter, who is in her twenties, if she's been taking her probiotics, because

apparently everyone needs to be babied by you now... awkward.
- You have no desire to get out of your pyjamas.
- A baby comes bursting out of your goulash. Or, in cases like my twins, thanks to an emergency C-section, out of your stomach, alien style. They usually don't strangle you afterwards, which is a nice feature.

Apparently some people considered my way to be negative. Well, I've got depression, so that's a bit like calling a shovel a shovel. It's not exactly great detective work to point out that I might be a tad negative. I have similar feelings about random people who point out the typos, spellos, and just plain wrongos in my writing. I'm dyslexic. You got me. How brilliant are you that you can point out errors in a dyslexic's tweet? Thank you for letting me know you think I'm stupid and won't communicate with me until I learn how to spell correctly. I don't like communicating with snobs anyway, so this saves us both a lot of trouble.... You smell like a putt. And you know exactly what I mean. I don't mean putt at all. I mean BUTT!

Having dyslexia and being a writer is an interesting thing. People constantly ask me how I can be a writer and be dyslexic. It's as if I constantly have to justify my existence. And to be honest, it is quite difficult for me to do so because I really don't understand why the question is asked in the first place. Dyslexia doesn't hinder my ability to think up interesting ideas. Dyslexia doesn't prevent me from imagining stories. Dyslexia doesn't mean that I cannot understand character, or plot, or structure. It simply means that what goes on in my brain can be a little jumbled when it comes out of my fingers. So? Why does that mean I can't write? I just have to take longer going over my stuff, and I have to hire an editor. But even people without dyslexia need an editor, so that really isn't a big deal. Same with reading: I might occasionally get held up and take longer in some areas, particularly when I'm tired, but I just work a bit harder. The way I see it, everybody has stuff they struggle with.

You don't just avoid all aspects of life because you have one issue. It would be like someone who had trouble kicking a ball, so they avoided anything that involved balls in any format. Not only would they refuse to play or watch football, but also basketball, tennis, or even lotto. They wouldn't use a fit ball in the gym. They couldn't use bath bombs. Now that seems a little over the top as a response to not being amazing at kicking a ball, doesn't it? Same with me avoiding writing just because I'm dyslexic. I love making up stories. I love communicating with people without the social anxiety of face-to-face contact. So why would I give up writing just because of dyslexia? You don't give up on something you love because of one minor problem; you work on it. And you don't give up on yourself because of one problem, like depression; you work on it. Kid, you'll move mountains.

Life Hacks for Women with PND

Before I end this book, I thought that I should give you some genuine tips to help deal with PND. Because as much as I try to put a sunny side to most things, I'm a smiling depressive—we tend to do that—but when you have PND, everyday chores and merely thinking can become an impossible task. Solutions that seem so simple to others are often drowned out by the barrage of negative critics inside our own heads. So I'd just like to give you some concrete things that you can grab hold of, because you've got enough going on right now without having to think about menial tasks. Here are seven tips to take the thinking right out of the equation, so you can get back to being the best you that you can be.

Tip 1: Outsource

I'd strongly recommend outsourcing support. PND does not occur in a vacuum, although it does seem very much as if you are trapped in the vacuum of space where no one can hear you scream. It is a whole family issue. Most women with PND are lacking support, whether it be an emotionally distant partner, dysfunctional family of origin, or having moved far away from family and friends. Women are often very much "alone" in some way. Hire a nanny or babysitter to fill that void. Nobody is Superwoman; everybody needs help. Even just four hours twice a week will have you feeling more in control. Use one day to sleep and the other to get things done.

Tip 2: Online Shopping

Try ordering food online. Sometimes doing big shopping trips is hard with a little one in tow. Managing to carry a baby or toddler or two plus heavy groceries can be a more strenuous workout than any *Zumba* class. Order big items online. There are, of course, always the big two companies in Australia, *Coles* and *Woolworths*, but other companies run delivery services as well, such as *Aussie Farmers Direct* and *Harris Farm*.

Tip 3: Use Electrical Goods

Get a dryer. Yep, you very well might feel like an environmental terrorist, but it will save you time. And right now time is precious to you. You don't need to be Enviro Woman every moment of your life. You can prioritise getting through the day for the next few years and then return to your ecologically friendly ways once you have the energy to smile, let alone lift your arms to hang washing.

Tip 4: Get Professional Help

Get a therapist. *Nice one, Sherlock, telling me to get a therapist. Obviously I know that, but where to start?* In Australia you can always check the list of Medicare Approved Providers in your area, call up, find out if they have a vacancy, and then see your GP to get a referral to that specific person. Or you can see your local GP and ask about a Mental Health Treatment Plan and ask who they would recommend you see. With a Mental Health Treatment Plan, Medicare Approved Providers give you either free or drastically discounted therapy. Other countries have similar websites with approved practitioners listed. Choose one in your area or go with your doctor's recommendation. And don't feel you have to stay with your therapist. If, after three sessions, they really don't seem to be getting you at all, try another one.

Medicare isn't the only organisation in Australia that helps with paying for psychologists. Both *BUPA* and *The Teacher's Health Fund* offer free one-on-one sessions with PIRI (Parent–Infant Research Institute) connected psychologists. Or at least they did when I was typing this. They might have changed; check with them. But with this service, there is no paying. Not even paying upfront and getting a refund. You simply show them your card, and they bill the Health Fund directly. I'm sure other Health Funds have similar setups. If you have private health insurance, then give them a call. They'll be able to send you information or recommend people. Don't be afraid to call. It's their job to help, and you're paying fees to get that help.

In Australia, your Child Health Nurse at your Community Centre can also refer you to see a social worker who can be of enormous benefit for pointing out options and strategies.

You might want to consider relationship counselling along with individual therapy. PND is a family issue. There is every chance that you may need relationship counselling with either your partner or ex-partner. Living with a person with depression can be tough on the partner, but living in a depressive state where you do not feel supported is also a harrowing situation. Both sides need to heal the rift, and a good place to start is a relationship therapist. In Australia, the organisation *Relationships Australia* is a national body that offers assistance with setting up and maintaining positive relationships in families and communities. Just call them up and ask them where to start. They're experts in the field, so don't worry if you don't have all the answers because that's what they're there to help you with.

If you've hit a breaking point, then it is time for serious intervention. There is no shame in needing more intensive help. It is far worse to make your children suffer through your increasingly self-destructive, and potentially dangerous, behaviours than it is to break the cycle and say, "I need serious help." Across Australia, there are Mother and Baby psychiatric units that allow you and your child/children, who is/are under one, to stay for treatment. They have nurses on staff to help with not only your care but also your baby's/babies'. They have psychiatrists and group therapists to assist you in healing. Speak to your GP about which mother-and-baby units are near you and how to access them. This level of intervention is not required by most sufferers of PND, but please don't be too ashamed to accept this help if you need it. You can be happy again.

Tip 5: Lamaze for Life

"Just breathe." Sometimes it seems like it's all too much and that you can't take it for a second longer. You have a baby crying, dishes piling up, and no help in sight. Just breathe. Everybody says it, but it does work. I find that I need a more structured approach to my breathing, than simply being told to take deep breaths. The use of tai-chi or chi-gung seems to be more helpful for me rather than simply taking deep breaths, as focusing on the instructions really allows me to detach for a moment, regain my energy, and start again. Even just a two-minute warm-up exercise can help, and the best bit is you can do it anywhere. If you have a toddler, they'll usually join in quite happily. Being a busy mum, you probably don't have time to dash out to a tai-chi class, but you can still learn the basics through an exercise DVD or even YouTube.

Tip 6: Keep a List

I also highly recommend keeping a list of contacts handy. A list of people and organisations to call if you are in a desperate state. You can even put them in an order of priority. In a moment of crisis, just grab the list and start at the beginning and don't stop until you've found someone who can help you. I have done this myself recently.

This year, I had a bad bout of gastro. I don't just tell you this because I have a shameless love of sharing my bowel movements with people—I mean, I do, but that's not the reason I'm mentioning it this time. This bout of gastro meant that I couldn't take my antidepressants. I simply couldn't keep them down, not to mention the husband is not exactly a quality nurse. He found it quite odd that I'd need to be checked in on more than twice a day, so dispensing medications was quite beyond him. I went from a Tuesday to Friday without any antidepressants. That's four days without antidepressants. What could go wrong in four days? Surely that's not that long. Wrong. The result of being off my antidepressants was swift and brutal. On the next Saturday, I was well enough to get out of bed and keep some food and water down. I was feeling very odd. I had been in a down phase for over six months prior to the gastro, but this was different. I took my antidepressant at about 8 am for the first time in four days and was thankfully able to keep it down, but it wasn't soon enough to stop the effects that the withdrawal had on me.

At 9 am that Saturday, I went back to bed. I still wasn't very well from four days of exploding from both ends and not being able to eat. I proceeded to have vivid nightmares of memories that I prefer to keep buried. There are some people that are of a theory that you must confront and deal with every single memory and feeling, but quite frankly, there are some that I'm perfectly happy with keeping buried deep down under the concrete fog of suppression. They can stay buried, as far as I'm concerned, because there are some things in this life that I will never be strong enough to deal with, and they get to stay in that box.

Unfortunately, they came leaping out of that box and began dancing around in my head. I woke up. They continued to run around unfettered. Jumping about, opening other boxes. I desperately tried to close them. I began to shake, I began to cry, and I began to think I was losing my mind. I felt that my kids would be better off without a crazy mother and that I should kill myself rather than have them endure my endless psychological burden on them. I tried to contact my husband; he was busy. I tried calling the medical centre my GP works at; they were fully booked, and nobody could see me. I then contacted my two best girlfriends, Helen and Lisa. They were probably busy; they've both got kids and commitments—Lisa was even in the process of publishing her book, *Destination Dachshund*—but they pretended they didn't. They sent me the number for a home-doctor visit and asked if there was someone they could call for me, someone they could get to come see me? They immediately wanted to look after me and make sure I was cared for. At this point, it was 11 am, and I sent the following message to my psychologist:

Hi ____. I'm really sorry to bother you on the weekend, but I'm slightly concerned that I might be having a bit of a psychological episode. I can't stop having nightmares, even when I'm awake. I think it is because I'm so depleted from gastro, which thankfully stopped, and I hadn't been able to keep my medication down since Tuesday and because the pain in my leg is quite bad at the moment but I'm really struggling and just don't quite know what I should do. I'd normally just duck in to see my GP, but she doesn't work on weekends, and nobody else can see me, and I was just unsure what I should do so was *wondering if you had any advice. Sorry, Robin.*

She sent me a message saying that she would call me back in 15 minutes.

In four hours, I had gone from feeling a vague sense of impending doom to feeling as if I was losing my mind and wanting to kill myself. Such a short amount of time and I was ready to end it. That's how intense sudden withdrawal from antidepressants can be. There was no lead-up into this overwhelming despair. It just hit full force within a matter of hours. I had started taking a new antidepressant a little over a month prior and had found it quite effective for me, but it was like all that had been undone, and I'd slid even further backwards.

When my psychologist called, she explained to me that I probably wasn't losing my mind and that I probably was suffering withdrawal symptoms. The feelings I was having were from the chemical imbalance rather than some sort of break in my mind. This was very comforting. She spoke to me for quite some time to make sure that I was okay and told me to go to the emergency department if I needed to and to not simply suffer through the symptoms if they were unbearable. That sudden withdrawal from medication was awful, but it would be over in a few days, and there were things that doctors could do for me in the interim, such as prescribe a drug like Xanax to keep me more settled whilst my regular medication kicked back in.

Just knowing that I wasn't crazy, that there was a reason that my brain seemed to be melting out of my ear, provided me with great relief. It gave me a lens to view my thoughts through that let me know that it would pass, and that they would go away. The symptoms were still present for me to cope with on my own, so I took Seroquel over the next few days whilst the worst side effects were present.

A week later and I was not only back to my "normal" self but I actually felt quite proud of myself. I know that probably sounds weird, proud of myself after having a complete meltdown, but I am. Two years ago, when I went into a psychiatric hospital, I was having similar feelings. I went to my husband for support—he's not good with the feelings—and he was too busy. I continued to flounder and could not cope and felt like there was nothing I could do. I kept on desperately not coping until a paediatrician at a hospital saw how much I was suffering when he was treating my sons and referred me to a social worker. This time round, in a matter of hours, I had repeated the same process— reached out to my husband; he was too busy, but I am hopeful that one day he will have made enough progress that he is willing to reach back during sickness or injury. On being rebuffed, I tried my GP. On being unsuccessful, I still didn't give up and contacted my two wonderful friends, Lisa and Helen, and then my psychologist.

In the last two years, I have made three fantastic decisions that have made me a stronger and better person. I chose Lisa and I chose Helen to be my friends—without them, my life would be so much less productive—and I picked the best psychologist that I have ever seen. Someone who understands me and how to treat me. Someone who is willing to take time out of their weekend to treat me. I am so proud of myself for making these healthy choices in my life. I am so proud that instead of spiralling out of control for months that I got onto it in a number of hours. Just because I fell yet again, didn't mean I couldn't get back up. And because of all that I have learned in these last couple of years, I was back up on my feet in record time. That's huge progress for me.

So seriously, keep a list of contacts. If in doubt, phone a friend, and also a professional. Friends can deal with some things, but major issues need professional intervention, and a true friend will remind you of that. That's the kind of friend you want at the top of your list. There are several organisations that will be happy for you to ring up and say, "I'm lost, I'm struggling, I need help, and I don't know what to do." They'll then ask you a whole bunch of questions in order to try to find out how best to help you. Answer them honestly so they can do their job.

It may feel intrusive, but you're worth it and you deserve help.

> In Australia, the main organisations are:
> **PANDA** http://www.panda.org.au/
> **PIRI** http://www.piri.org.au/
> **Black Dog Institute**
> http://www.blackdoginstitute.org.au/
> **Lifeline** https://www.lifeline.org.au/
> **Gidget Foundation:**
> http://gidgetfoundation.com.au/

I am in no way affiliated with any of these organisations. I'm barely affiliated with myself. And my listing of these organisations doesn't mean that they approve of me or even know anything about me. I'm simply listing them because they are the major bodies associated with the areas of depression and anxiety that will be able to give you more specific advice. I'm not a professional; I'm just a mad cow.

Tip 7: Auto Respond

I'd also consider having a bank of responses to things people commonly say if they find out that you have postnatal depression. Sometimes it can be hard to respond appropriately in the moment when someone cracks out a deeply personal question or a hurtful stereotype, so it's often best if you have something ready to go so that you can just be on autopilot. I have prepared a list of my super helpful responses to questions I commonly get. There's a slight possibility that you might want to think of your own.

You can't have postnatal depression. You like your baby.

Response: Yes, you can. Piss off.

The vast majority of the women I have met who are battling postnatal depression, both in and out of the chicken coup, absolutely love their kids. They sing to their children, they hug them, they praise them, they play with them, they pick them up, and they do everything a "normal" loving mother would do. Despite all this love, they still struggle with anxiety and coping. When your baby is unsettled, that's stressful for anyone. Most people care if their baby screams; however, once the crisis is over, most mums can start to calm down also. It is tough, it is unpleasant, and they look forward to when this phase will pass and their tension can ease.

With a mum with PND, our thoughts spiral out of control—I've done something to upset the baby, it's my fault the baby is upset, I'll never be able to soothe my baby, I'm a terrible mother, I'm ruining my precious baby's life and causing permanent damage because I can't work out what is wrong, I'm a terrible person, I'm useless, I'm worthless, the baby would be better off without me so that they could get a better mother. The crisis is over, but the thoughts keep churning around in our heads. With every unsettled period and every perceived mistake we make, the thoughts we have regarding ourselves and our fitness to parent our beautiful child become darker. Tears come, screams escape, and zoning out happens. As a result of this seemingly uncontrollable negative thinking, many mums like myself become paralysed by guilt.

We love our baby so much that we drive our bodies and minds to ruin making superhuman efforts to be perfect. Consequently, our body breaks down, and we can no longer function. For others, they become so lost in the nightmare in their head that they start to retreat and zone out.

They are physically present but not mentally. They can have some bonding issues simply because they checked out of reality because it was more painful than disliking their babies. And yes, there are a few that start to resent their baby for dredging up all these feelings, and this resentment can start to spiral into anger and hate. It can seriously affect the mother-child bond. But from my experience, the angst ridden, tearful, making-yourself-sick kind of postnatal depression seems far more prevalent. Regardless of how it manifests, it is highly treatable, and people do get better with help. They can shed these negative thoughts and become the happy, positive parents that they want to be.

Oh my god! Have you been thinking about hurting your baby?

Response: Nope, but I'm thinking about hurting someone right now.

Not everyone with PND wants to hurt their baby. Left untreated and unsupported, it could get to these extreme levels but generally no. Women with PND are far more likely to hate themselves than their babies. They feel hopeless and useless and think that their baby and the world in general would be better off without them. But of course, not all women with PND have suicidal idealisations. It isn't a stereotypical, one-size-fits-all condition. Suffering from depression does not automatically make you psychotic or dissociative. It's actually quite offensive to treat someone actively getting treatment as if they're completely unhinged and are on the verge of a murder-suicide at any moment. And treating people as if they can't be trusted actually holds up treatment and makes people unwilling to communicate because they'll have to put up with a whole host of bullshit assumptions.

You still have your sense of humour, so everything must be ok.
Response: Oh, does that mean that you're not okay? Because you're not particularly funny.

When I was being carted away in the ambulance with full-blown pancreatitis, I was still making jokes. The mask of humour in public stays firmly in place, lest I turn into a gibbering mess in public and become a social outcast. I'm what is known as a smiling depressive—you'll rarely see one of us without our smile mask on.

You look good, so you must be okay.
Response: Thank you. I'm one sexy bitch.

Looks can be deceiving. People get food poisoning all the time when eating something they thought looked delicious.

Everybody feels like that.
Response: Oh fuck, it's not a competition.

True, every mother has moments like this, but the feelings don't last as long. Minimising these long-term, pervasive feelings only keeps a woman from getting help. It doesn't help.

Some people are just more anxious than others; you don't need treatment.

Response: But I don't want to be as unpleasant to be around as you are.

You do not have to live with anxiety. You deserve a better life and so do your kids. Some people may be happy to live as a shaking anxious mess and have those they love suffer through this, but that doesn't make it right, and it doesn't mean you don't deserve help. Anxiety is very treatable.

Other people have it tougher than you, so why aren't you coping?
Response: Hooray for them.

Seriously, good on them. If you're going to compare, do it properly. Do they have your history?—have they had your health complaints?—do they get more help? And even if they are this amazing superhuman who can juggle 17 kids without breaking a sweat, whilst working full time, without any babysitting, and have perfectly well-adjusted children, it doesn't mean you're a bad person for not coping. Everybody is different. We all have different skills and have had different role models. It's okay to struggle with things and for others to find it easy. We aren't all scientific geniuses, and we aren't all amazing singers. It's okay to have your own skills and your own struggles, and it's okay to get help with areas you struggle with. Some people sail through their children's newborn years and then struggle once they're teenagers; others do the reverse. It's okay to be different.

You're a selfish mother and just want to do your own thing and not tend your baby?
Response: Fuck off.

No real follow-up needed on that one.

Just keep going and it will get better.
Response: Sure, and if you just keep walking on a broken leg, it will get better too… sure, it will…

Because mental illness is largely invisible, people feel as if they can just ignore it, and it will go away. Not all health issues work that way. You can ignore a cold, but you can't ignore a gunshot wound.

In short, get yourself a trusted team of professionals. Don't just trust the first therapist that comes by. I could seriously write a whole book on therapists I have had failed relationships with. All of whom I continued to turn up and pay money to because I was too embarrassed to leave. I didn't want to be rude, so I kept on going and wasting my time and money. Don't do that; get the right one for you. If your therapist isn't working out for you, then go try another one and another one and another one until you find the right one for you. Don't be afraid to outsource help. Sometimes paid help is actually even better than family because they're reliable, with no strings attached. Obviously check them out and all—don't just hire a random off the street—but don't think needing help makes you a failure. Everybody needs help. And keep a list of contacts to work through in a crisis. Make sure that you have good friends on that list. The kinds of friends who will tell you what you need to hear, not just fob you off and try to distract you or dismiss your feelings. You are important, and you are worth getting help for.

Memoir from the Madhouse

And now it is time to bid you adieu. Thanks for bearing with me. I thought, what better way to end this book than giving you an insight into how I have been using writing to help me process my feelings and experiences around postnatal depression? I have already shared with you how I used fiction to cope with my daughter's hip dysplasia, so it's only fitting that I actually show you what I have been working on in regards to the topic that we've been discussing. On exiting hospital, I began working on a memoir about my time in the madhouse. But I found I had so many ideas and stimulation that a standard memoir wasn't going to be enough for the scope of what I felt. It would get out the information but not the feelings. So I switched to doing what they call "true fiction." Which is a made-up story that is realistic. I took my experiences from that time, the rest of my life, conversations I have overheard, things I have seen, articles I have read, essentially everything and everyone that has ever passed through my life, merged them all into one conglomerate blob, and started writing a fictional project called *Memoir from the Madhouse*. So kick back, relax, and enjoy some fiction. Well, it gets a bit dark, so "enjoy" might not be the right word. Read it anyway?

I am running, running faster than I've ever run before. The cold from the dewy ground runs up my bare legs and covers my naked body with goose pimples. But still, I run on. The warmth is fleeting, the wind is chasing me, and they are hunting me. I run naked in the cold dark night, and all the while, I think, *I'm not crazy, I'm not crazy.*

Out of my periphery, I see a nurse approach. I let out a delirious laugh and keep on running.

"Run, run, run as fast as you can..."

The wind whips away my words, and I still run on. The ground starts to gently slope downwards, and in the darkness, I lose my bearings. I trip. I roll. Arms and legs flail at impossible angles. The world slows down as sky and earth blur into one. I smile and think about what has brought me here, starkers, in the dead of night, chasing demons, in the psychiatric hospital's grounds.

6 Hours Earlier

I sit in Consultation Room 2, staring at my psychiatrist. I have no idea what he is saying. His voice is so soft that I can only make out every second sentence if I'm lucky. Regardless, I nod as if I understand. I don't want him to think I'm rude or worse, stupid. My constantly interrupting to say, "Eh?" or, "What?" only results in him repeating his mumbles anyway. So instead, I just nod along as if I agree.

"Are you anxious about going home tomorrow?" Finally a sentence I can hear.

"No," I lie.

Of course I'm anxious. I've got newborn twins and a two year old. They're hard work. I have to somehow keep on functioning, no, mumctioning, despite the fact that the twins won't sleep, which means I can't sleep either. All work and no sleep makes Aydan a dull girl. Perhaps they could be trained to settle one another. One cries, and the other rubs their back, then they roll over and swap jobs. That'd be pretty sweet, but although I'm in the nuthouse, even I know that won't happen.

"Really?" my psychiatrist raises an eyebrow. "Last time you were supposed to go home, you had such an anxiety attack that we had to transfer you to a medical hospital. A month ago, you wanted to commit suicide."

I shrug. More words are spoken that I nod thoughtfully along too. God only knows what I've agreed to in these sessions.

"Do you like cap guns and pillows?" Nods in agreement.

"Do you still wet the bed?" Nods thoughtfully.

"Do you have a Christ complex?" Nods politely.

"Do you like the smell of your own farts?" Nods vigorously.

He probably thinks I'm the biggest psycho to ever have graced this Crackpot's with Babies Unit. No doubt I've inadvertently agreed to having a fetish for gingerbread men, having partaken in cock fighting as a chicken, and having to burp three times every time I hear the word "purple," lest the world ends. So it's not surprising that Doctor Huang is so shocked by my casual attitude.

Truth be told, I'm just quietly packing shit. My husband and I have arranged for a babysitter to come for a few hours a day during baby rush hour. From four to seven o'clock sucks with the under threes. They're cranky, they need baths, they need dinner, and they need to go to bed. Times that by three, and I seriously struggle. The babysitter coming at these times doesn't help me rest. Just helps me make sure none of my kids are neglected. I want to rest. We can't afford rest. Fucking money.

"A lot can change in a month."

4 Weeks Earlier

My husband pulls into the small parking lot. I stare straight ahead at the even brick wall before me. Old red brick. Perfectly ordered. Nothing can penetrate it. It's a complete barrier between the psychiatric hospital and the rest of the world. It's so blank. Just evenly spaced red blocks.

"We're here," my husband announces the obvious. "Should we get your stuff and go in?"

"I don't want to go in." I turn to my husband, tears welling in my eyes. "I want to stay with you."

He sighs. He does that a lot of late. He stares up at the grey roof of our car and closes his eyes for a moment, as if trying to will this whole situation to disappear. He stretches his neck from side to side before turning to stare at me.

"You wanted to go here; you thought that this would be a good idea."

"I've changed my mind." Tears begin to fall.

"You have to go." He sighs again.

"Don't you want me to stay with you?" I desperately want some sign that he still loves me.

"Of course I do." He's no longer looking at me but staring at the bricks in front of us. He rolls his eyes. And sighs for a third time.

"So, let's go back home."

"No." He shakes his head. "You said you were going so you have to go."

I am about to protest, but one of the twins in the back starts to make noises. I look back at my perfect babies; they smile back. I can't help but break into a grin in return. They're too cute. Once they have teeth, toothpaste companies will be beating down the door to offer them advertising contracts. My husband uses the distraction to get out of the car.

"We're going on a little holiday," I say with forced enthusiasm. They can't understand a word that I'm saying, but I feel the need to explain things anyway. "Daddy's just going to set up the pram, and then we'll head in. It'll be an adventure."

My husband opens up the back door behind the driver's seat and unclips the car capsule from its base to put it onto the pram. I get out of the car and do the same with the remaining twin. They look so cute in their little capsules, snuggled up under blankets. I immediately want to grab them out and hug them, but that's not very practical. My husband starts walking off with the boys. He's got his suit on. Ready to head to work once I'm checked in, he must already be in a business frame of mind. Take no prisoners, charge ahead.

"I haven't got my bags yet," I tell his back.

"I thought I'd grab them once we knew exactly where your room would be," he replies. His face is expressionless. He may as well be talking about dropping me off at the library rather than for three weeks at a psychiatric hospital for all the emotion he is expressing.

"Good plan," I say, giving him what I hope is a cheeky grin. I want to crack that cold facade of his. "Leave my bags in the car with the engines running just in case we need to make a quick getaway."

His shoulders sag as he sighs yet again.

"Well, if you're gonna be like that, I'll just get them now," he mutters, swinging the pram around and heading back to the car.

I frown. He was supposed to laugh. He was supposed to change his mind, pack us all back into the car, and rescue me.

The husband opens the boot and dumps one bag into the bottom of the pram and swings the other one onto his shoulder. He looks at me, then turns to the boot and slams it with a grunt. I shudder a little. He's mad at me; I don't like it when he's mad at me.

"Come on, I've gotta get to work," he says as he pushes the pram past me and towards the entryway.

I rush to catch up with him.

"That's nice," I say, pointing at a statue of the Virgin Mary. I'm trying to make conversation and am hoping to appeal to his Catholic background.

"Pretty standard," he grunts back, "nothing special."

If I'd been Catholic, I would have known this wouldn't have worked as a conversation piece. I look down at the ground as I follow along.

"I guess this is where we go in." My husband has stopped the pram.

I look up; the red brick has stopped, and the entire front is now shiny glass, outlined with pristine white slabs of concrete. It looks almost like the entrance to a hotel rather than what I expected from a psychiatric hospital. I was expecting more old red brick, maybe some cracked concrete, and the odd bloodstain from all the escape attempts. This all looks very civilised. I nod dumbly, and we walk through the large automated glass doors.

The quietness hits me. It is very still. One woman sits behind a large wooden counter, looking every bit like a receptionist at a big hotel, and not at all like a cranky psych nurse desperate for a cigarette break. The area is open with well-kept blue carpet. An indoor garden is to my right, and there are seats set around it. A few people sit there quietly talking. I can hear nothing but a gentle murmur and the trickle of the irrigation system. We must have somehow gotten lost and walked too far. It didn't seem as if we walked for long.

"Are we in the right place?" I ask my husband, confused.

I can't hear any tortured howls, and everybody is walking around in regular clothes. There isn't a straitjacket in sight. No orderlies appear to be roaming about, ready to tackle dissidents, either. There is nothing psychiatric hospitaly about this place at all. There has to be some mistake.

"I'll go ask," my husband mutters and wanders off to the lady at the counter.

I move over to the pram and coo at my smiley boys. They're looking at me with such love in their eyes that I immediately regret sucking so badly that I can't cope with them. My daughter's eyes looked at me with that same amount of love when I dropped her off at preschool this morning. I press my hand to my chest in an attempt to physically stop the pain burning there.

"She told us to wait over there." So caught up in my thoughts I hadn't even noticed my husband return.

"Is it because I'm crying?"

He shrugs. "Maybe."

I follow him to a somewhat secluded section in the foyer. I hadn't noticed it on arrival, as it is hidden off to the side by clever use of potted plants and support beams. I try to wipe away my tears discreetly. I don't want to bring anymore shame to myself or to him. He hates any hint of emotion so tears are far too much. There are padded burgundy chairs in the enclave. I take a seat. My husband avoids the seat next to me and sits across from me instead. He doesn't even want to be near me.

"I don't want to go," I say pleadingly to him.

He tries to put on a smile. It is shaking under the strain.

"It'll be okay," he says. "It'll be for the best. How else will you get better?"

My peripheral vision begins fading; the world is going dark.

"I don't want to be locked up in here." I begin to physically curl up, unable to stop myself from showing my internal agitation. "I don't want to be alone."

32 Years Ago

It is dark. I am awake. I am being yelled at. I am wet. Where am I? It is Dad. He is yelling. He is always yelling. Ouch. He is smacking. Where am I? What is wrong? I am in his bed. Why am I in his bed? I am alone with him. I hate him. I hate being alone with him. Why am I alone with him? I must have fallen asleep with Mum, and she has left. Now I am alone with him, and he is yelling. I am cold frightened and wet. He is ripping my pants off and yelling.

"You fucking filthy animal. You fucking pissed in my fucking bed. What the fuck is wrong with you, you fucking piece of shit."

I am in trouble. I wiggle and scream and try to get away. I want my pants. I don't want to have no pants and be with him. He grabs me and holds me down in the wetness.

"If you're gonna piss everywhere like an animal, then I'm gonna treat you like a fucking animal."

I try to get up, but he pushes my face back down into my wee. He grabs me by the throat and starts yelling some more. I can't understand what he is saying. He is just yelling. He shakes me and throws me back on the bed. I try to get up to run away, but he grabs me. I have to get out. I don't want to be alone in the dark with no pants with Dad. I scream, I struggle; I am suffocating, I am blacking out. I can't breathe. I will not fail. I will escape. I bite. I bite hard. I bite down on the hand across my mouth with all that I can. I taste blood.

"You fucking cunt."

He grabs me by the hair. He drags me. He is dragging me away. I want my pants. I don't want to have no pants. I need my pants. He throws me into the nightmare room. It is scary there. It is dark. There is no light. I am afraid of the dark. He shuts the door.

"You can fucking stay there, you fucking animal."

I am scared. I am alone. I cry. I try to get out. I open the door. Pain. Blinding pain. My fingers have been slammed in the door.

"I knew you'd try to get out, you sneaky fucking cunt. You fucking stay in there, or I will kill you."

I cry, I cry, I cry. I am so lonely. I am scared. I want my doll to keep me safe from the nightmares.

"Aydan?" I hear my brother's voice. It is magic. It is safe. I am happy. "Are you okay?"

"I am scared. I want my doll."

"Okay, I'll get it. I'll sneak it to you. Just give me a minute."

I wait. I see a crack of light under the door. I watch it and wait. Soon, that light will bring me my brother and my doll. I will be okay. Big brother is here. The crack widens, and I see my brother's hand and my doll. I reach for the doll. Suddenly screaming. The hand and the doll are disappearing.

"You fucking cunt. You think you're smarter than me? Gonna be the big man and make all the decisions? I will fucking end you." I hear a loud thud.

"She just wants her doll. I wasn't letting her out again. I was just giving her her doll."

"You never fucking learn, do you? I fucking put her in there, and she'll fucking stay in there until I say so. If I want her to have a doll, I'll give her a fucking doll. I decide what to do."

"But she's scared."

Another thud.

"She just wants her doll because she's scared of the dark." The voice is getting lower and more unsteady.

"That's why she's fucking in there, isn't it? She won't fucking wet the bed again if she's too scared to. She's fucking three years old! She shouldn't be wetting the bed."

More thuds. Silence. I wait. I stare at the light under the door. I lie on the ground and stare under the door. Big Brother is lying there.

"Hello?" There is no answer. "Big Brother? Are you okay?" His body twitches a little, but there is no answer. Dad has made him too sick to be able to speak or move again.

I crawl away from the door. It is not a nice light anymore. It is marred by Big Brother's sad body.

I move into the corner of the nightmare, away from the light. It is cold. It is dark. I am alone. I am afraid. I close my eyes. I am rocking. Someone is rocking me. I am safe. I open my eyes. In the distance I can see a castle. It is so dark that I can barely make it out, but it is there. The goblin with its arms around me pats my head soothingly.

"Come, dear one. We must go to your palace."

"My palace?"

"Yes, dear one. Your palace awaits. All the woodland creatures are there waiting to protect you."

I smile. I get up and walk to the palace, hand in hand with my goblin. It is dark. I am alone. I am safe. I am the queen.

4 Weeks Ago

"Aydan?"

I snap back to attention. How long had I been daydreaming for? I stare at my husband, and he is in turn staring at the source of the voice. A middle-aged woman with a sensible brown bob is smiling warmly at me. The admittance nurse is here. Oh God, it's really happening. Nobody is coming to save me. It's all real now.

Hopefully I can get *Memoir from the Madhouse* cleaned up enough one day to publish for you as well. At the moment, it seems to reflect the ever-changing environment that is my brain and keeps evolving and morphing. And the title keeps on changing. I can't even lock onto a title, ugh. Even now I'm thinking, "Wouldn't *Based on a True Story* be a better title?" But please know that if you have ever had these thoughts, you are not alone. I was there and periodically go back there. It's okay.

Depression is really tough, but you're tougher. You have already gotten this far, and you're not alone, because I'm here too. You can join my girl tribe. We can do this.

Other Titles by Robin Elizabeth

The following titles are available in ebook only. Please check your favourite ebook retailers to see if they have a copy, or check out http://riedstrap.wordpress.com for more information.

What Happens in Book Club (E1): It's Not Me; It's You
What Happens in Book Club (E2): I'm Just Not That Into You
What Happens in Book Club (E3): It's Complicated

About Bookends Publishing

Bookends Publishing is a new Australian consultancy publisher. It came into being to help authors achieve their publishing dreams, provide publication advice to indie authors and opportunities for new, emerging, and established writers.

In 2017, the Bookends Australian Writing Award will be established to showcase Australian writers and their many talents. All shortlisted and winning entries will be published in an anthology.

http://bookendspublishing.com.au

www.ingramcontent.com/pod-product-compliance
Lightning Source LLC
Chambersburg PA
CBHW032037290426
44110CB00012B/847